WHY DOCTORS SKIP BREAKFAST

Wellness Tips to Reverse Aging, Treat Depression, and Get a Good Night's Sleep

D1519752

GREGORY CHARLOP, MD

CONTENTS

PREFACE   1

CHAPTER 1: WELLNESS AND OPTIMAL HEALTH   4

CHAPTER 2: IS AGING PREVENTABLE?   26

CHAPTER 3: HOW TO REVERSE AGING   39

PART I - FOOD   39

PART II - SUPPLEMENTS, MEDICATIONS, AND LABS 59

PART III - LIFESTYLE, TECHNOLOGY, AND WELLNESS

77

CHAPTER 4: THE BEST SLEEP OF YOUR LIFE   106

CHAPTER 5: SLEEP AND ELITE PERFORMERS   138

CHAPTER 6: DEPRESSION AND THE KETAMINE
    REVOLUTION   147

CHAPTER 7: PUTTING IT ALL TOGETHER   165

ABOUT THE AUTHOR   177

REFERENCES   178

Preface

Life starts early in the operating room. I arrive by 6 a.m., change into hospital scrubs, and head into the sterile surgical suite. Nurses clad in blue caps and masks wheel scalpels and supplies down the hall.

As an anesthesiologist, I ferry my patients into a drug-induced twilight, detached from the world. Their body systems, from breathing to heartbeat, are under my control. With powerful medications, I switch off their brains in preparation for surgery. They are free of pain, fear, and distress. Patients have no memory of surgery, yet retain everything that makes them, them.

Time to prepare

I survey the ventilators, pumps, and monitors that I'll use to keep my patients alive and flip switches to activate their self-test sequences. The machines hum and flicker to life.

With my fingerprint, I unlock the secure medication supply cabinet. One by one, each of the drawers open to reveal syringes, needles, masks, and tubes. I examine the tiny glass drug bottles I'll use to treat pain, regulate blood pressure, respond to emergencies, numb nerves, and alter consciousness.

Under the cold fluorescent lights of the OR, I snap the top off of a medication vial and puncture the black rubber stopper. A milky-white fluid fills the syringe. After drawing up the proper dose of each drug, I label everything and arrange my tray.

I'm ready.

Back at the main desk, I pull up a chair next to the computer terminal to review my upcoming cases one final time, savoring black coffee as I read. I enjoy these quiet moments just before the day officially begins.

Surgeons, anesthesiologists, and a variety of other doctors walk past the control desk with their stethoscopes and white coats. These physicians, my colleagues, trained at some of the country's top institutions. Harvard, Princeton, Stanford, and MIT. They've published papers, led departments, and saved countless lives. They're the best of the best.

The preoperative suite buzzes with life as the nurses prepare the first patients of the day. They check blood sugars, complete forms, and answer questions.

Down the hall, a young lady anxiously awaits surgery to cure her breast cancer. An elderly man chats with his family before heading into joint surgery. Advanced age ravaged his bones, robbing him of his ability to walk. Thanks to a recent medical breakthrough, he'll soon be able to leave his wheelchair without pain. And a young boy, already sedated with our special "happy juice," giggles with his parents before his upcoming hernia repair.

The surgeons sit near me, sipping coffee. We discuss the day's plans with the charge nurse and the anesthesia team. Today should be a good day.

Scattered across the control desk are books, files, surgical glasses, computers, briefcases, and coffee mugs. But there is no food to be found. While the java flows like a river, almost all of these remarkable doctors skip breakfast.

The room is full of distinguished surgeons preparing to go into battle for 10, 12, 14 hours, yet they choose to start the day on an empty stomach.

Why? What do these doctors know?

That's the story of this book. I will introduce you to the new world of wellness medicine. We'll shatter old myths that are quietly ruining your life and show you the path to vibrant health.

Breakfast is not the most important meal of the day. Aging is reversible. We can treat depression, even when conventional medications have failed. And, a great night of sleep is easier than you think.

Let's get started.

Chapter 1

Wellness and Optimal Health

Jack grew up in the business. His mother was a famous actress and his father was a successful movie producer. Following in his family's footsteps, Jack pursued a life in the entertainment industry as a writer and director.

A hard worker, Jack was at his desk at five each morning powering through a script. He ate breakfast at seven with other industry bigshots and spent the rest of the day at the studio. After work, he'd hit the Hollywood bar scene and hobnob with young starlets. Jack was the toast of the town.

Life was good.

As with so many others in Hollywood, his success didn't last long. A year into his thriving career, the wheels started coming off. He gained weight and wasn't sleeping well. His nights were restless and his days lacked focus. His productivity dropped. While he once churned out script after script, now he could barely finish a scene. His mood darkened and he stopped getting invites to the best parties. Nobody wanted to be around a sour and irritable person in career freefall.

Even worse, his energy level fell. Imperceptible at first, his fatigue gradually worsened until he was unable to maintain his daily work schedule. One evening, while driving home from the studio after another disappointing day, he fell asleep at the wheel and crashed his Porsche into a tree. Thankfully, nobody was hurt.

That was the moment Jack realized that he had to turn his life around.

A New Day

Your alarm goes off, but you don't need it. You're already awake and full of energy to tackle the morning. You spring out of bed, do a few pushups to get the blood pumping, and take a quick cold shower. You head to the kitchen to brew a fresh cup of black coffee and then you're off to win the day.

You go out and land a new deal, knowing that you're powered with enough stamina and self-confidence to get the job done.

After work, you hit the gym or enjoy an invigorating run. You play with your kids and go out to dinner with friends. You're living the life of your dreams.

When you have energy, vitality and health, you have it all.

What is wellness?

I'm going to say it. Western medicine has the wrong goal. Our focus is off.

Go into any doctor's office and all they'll talk about are individual diseases, abnormal lab values, and medications. They'll discuss your potassium levels, weight, and temperature. They will plot you on curves and zero in on individual organs. They're looking for a problem to treat with a drug.

We mistakenly key in on little issues and abnormalities rather than the whole person. Doctors are constantly putting out fires rather than trying to make you (to borrow a phrase) better, stronger, and faster.

In other words, the goal of medicine is to repair breaks

rather than to make someone more vibrant and alive.

To be sure, there is a role for treating individual diseases. If you have an infection, require surgery (and anesthesia) or your thyroid level is low, you need traditional medical care. After all, I am a doctor and I know the power of medicine to fix even the most complex problems.

My objection to healthcare is that we set our sights too low. We shouldn't limit ourselves to fixing what's broken. Rather, our aim should be to reach our maximum potential. We should optimize our bodies and minds so we can live our best lives.

To me, that's what wellness is all about. Wellness isn't the absence of disease. Just because your kidneys are working properly and your blood pressure is 120/80, that doesn't mean you're well. Wellness means that you feel strong and vital. You're ready to face the world head-on. You have force, focus, and vigor.

Wellness means that you feel good about being you.

Imagine waking up powerful with the energy to tackle the day. More drive, sharper thinking, and a better mood. Who doesn't want to feel more vibrant and alive?

Do you struggle to get out of bed in the morning? Do you feel like you aren't doing as well at work as you'd like? Do you wrestle with feelings of sadness and self-doubt? Are you insecure? Is your body where you'd like it to be? Are you growing old before your time? Is it hard for you to stay focused? Have you lost interest in relationships?

Wellness is your answer.

Wellness will uplift your body and mind. By focusing on you as a whole person, we can unleash your power. This book shows you how.

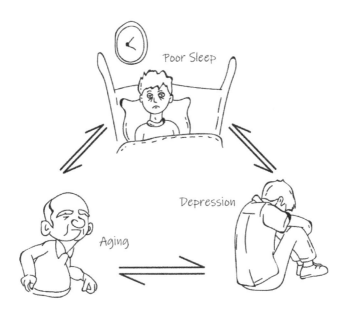

Aging, poor sleep, and depression are all related

Why fall short?

You don't need to live with the ordinary. You can do better.

The modern science of wellness will give you the keys to unlock your full potential and open doors to a successful new career, meaningful relationships, and a life filled with excitement.

You'll face your job with renewed energy and creativity. When you feel healthier and more energized, you'll be on your way to promotions and accolades. You'll be more creative. Coworkers will gravitate toward you and your positive attitude. Unlike Jack, you'll develop the right habits to achieve and maintain success.

Folks want to be around other happy, bright people. When your colleagues determine who should spearhead an important project, they'll naturally pick you. They'll see your vitality and self-confidence and naturally trust you to get the job done.

You score win after win. Before long, you'll be flooded with promotions and new job offers. Why would anyone want to work with a tired cynic when they can team up with you?

Aging

Quick: what comes to mind when you think of older peple? Low energy, dementia, depression, and frailty? Do you believe that a nursing home is inevitable?

I have some major news for you. The science is out, and aging is a disease, not a destiny. In other words, all the stuff we think of as aging doesn't need to happen to you. Sure, you'll grow older chronologically, but you don't need to accumulate the serious illnesses and chronic diseases we associate with the aged.

How can this be? Since aging is itself a disease, it can be prevented. With the right mixture of diet, sleep, supplements, and medication, you can ward off the disease of aging and enjoy vibrant health and energy well into your later years.

Rather than spend your 70s, 80s, and even 90s riddled with illness, you can enjoy those decades. Start a new career, travel, and spend quality time with family. You can literally gain decades of quality life by reversing the ravages of time. In the next chapter, we'll review the science of aging. Then, we'll explain how to stay young.

What's holding you back?

If you're reading this book, you have great potential. Besides obviously having good taste, you have a desire to live your best life. You want success, happiness, wealth, self-esteem, and strong relationships. You have goals.

What's keeping you from being your best self?

Where does that low energy, self-doubt, or brain fog come from?

A variety of malevolent factors may be keeping you from living the life of your dreams. Poor diet, depression, and lack of sleep are conspiring against you.

Together we'll explore what's robbing you of the life that you deserve.

You don't want to burn out and squander a promising career as Jack did. He was able to turn his life around, and so can you. Now is your time to fight back and regain control of your health, wealth, and energy.

Protection from infection

In addition to your body and mind, we want to energize your immune system. A strong immune system will help protect you from dangerous infections like COVID-19, pneumonia, and the flu.

If left unchecked, aging, sleep deprivation, and depression weaken the immune system. Over time, some of your body's warrior white blood cells will become senescent (see below) and ineffective. Proper sleep and other techniques outlined in this book will revitalize your immune system, reverse senescence, and help protect you from infections like the coronavirus.

You are what (and when) you eat

You make small decisions every day that shape your future. What's for dinner? Will you have a snack? Should you eat breakfast?

Eat right, and you will enjoy power and focus. Eat poorly, and you'll age prematurely. Surprisingly, when you eat is almost as important as what you eat. All it takes are a few small mistakes to set your day back. The wrong foods at the wrong time are all it takes to drain you of vitality.

The great news is that you don't need to eat broccoli all day to achieve the life you desire. We'll review the secrets to a healthy diet in chapter 3.

Depression

Depression can strike anyone. While it's normal to experience temporary grief from the loss of a job or loved one, some people suffer from severe clinical depression. People with clinical depression often lose interest in formerly pleasurable activities, feel hopeless, and lack energy. Depression can last for years and has no obvious cause.

Clinical depression can be devastating. To those suffering from depression, the day holds little interest and tomorrow looks bleak. While some depressed people maintain successful careers and beautiful families, their illness robs them of the joy in life. Simple tasks—like climbing out of bed in the morning—can be monumental struggles.

While there are a lot of pills and therapies for depression, most aren't very effective. Sadly, many people are forced to take antidepressant medication every day with little to show other than unwanted side effects.

Thankfully, there is now a novel and highly effective treatment for depression: ketamine. As an expert in this powerful medication, I'll show how you might benefit from its remarkable antidepressant effects. Ketamine can often cure depression, even when other treatments have failed. We'll also take a look at how food, nutrition, and cognitive behavioral therapy might help. If you or someone you love suffers from depression, read on. We'll discuss depression in greater detail in chapter 6.

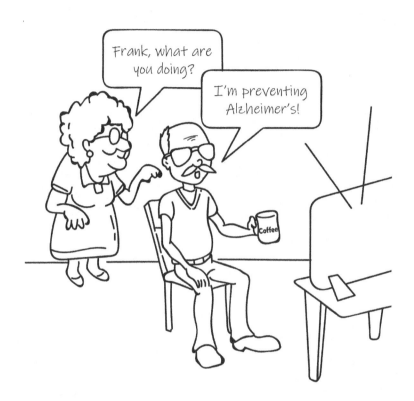

Coffee will perk you up

Here's the great news. One of the easiest things you can do for your health doesn't involve the gym, kale, or sacrifice.

In fact, you don't need to give anything up or break a sweat.

All you need to do is drink (more) coffee. You read that right. One of America's favorite drinks is also one of the healthiest. With each cup, you'll enjoy more energy, focus, and health. The natural antioxidants, oils, caffeine, and nutrients in your cup of Joe will help prevent depression, diabetes, and Alzheimer's disease.

There's some exciting new scientific research on this wonder food I'll share with you in chapter 3. We'll look at how much you should drink and when. Read on, and toast to your health.

Imagine the potential

I'm here to tell you that you don't need to settle. There's no reason that you should suffer through life with a mediocre career. If your goal is to create a company, rise to CEO, publish a new book, become a doctor, star in a movie, turn heads as a model, or give back to your community through charity, you deserve the energy and vitality to get the job done.

Don't come home at the end of the day too tired to work out, play with your kids, or spend quality time with your partner. You can unlock true stamina and get the most out of life.

Career, family, friends, charity, and self-care. Once you're healthy and the clouds of depression and self-doubt lift, you really can have it all.

In this book, we'll take a close look at what's robbing you of your energy and draining your vitality. One by one, we'll give you the roadmap to turn back the clock on aging, fight depression, improve your sleep, increase your focus, boost your energy, and unlock your potential.

This book is full of tips you can easily do at home like diet, fasting, strategic caffeine, and proper sleep techniques. Together, we'll examine some cutting-edge medical interventions like ketamine, metformin, and sleep apnea treatment. We'll look at some of the coolest medical gizmos and wearable technology and explore how you can use them to get an edge. And we will make a list of labs you need to evaluate and optimize your health.

This book will give you a clear pathway to unlock your full potential.

Treatment must be customized

We all know someone like this. Let's call her Jane. Jane can eat pizza every day. She has dessert with each meal and is never one to pass on seconds. Her only exercise is walking to and from her car. Yet, she's thin, energetic, and always smiling. When she goes to her doctor for her annual checkup, everything looks great. She even has perfect eyesight.

Unfortunately, most of us are not like Jane.

We all come to the table with our own slate of medical problems and past dietary habits. But even beyond visible illnesses like diabetes or liver disease, we are different at the cellular level. Just as two people might respond to the stress of public speaking differently—one relishing the limelight while the other runs in fear—our bodies are designed to react differently to stresses at the microscopic level.

Our genetic material, our DNA, is one of a kind. Each of us has slightly different versions of enzymes and proteins. Therefore, we react to chemical and physiologic stresses differently. Some substances that are harmless to Jane might be toxic for you. She may make a bag of chips disappear without a trace, while you'll gain weight just from looking at a potato.

We're all different.

While this book will examine the latest science you can use to fight aging, improve your mood, and strengthen your energy levels, not every technique will work equally for everybody. We're all unique and each of our bodies will react differently to challenges and treatment.

While we will share tips and tricks that will benefit everyone, you'll need to focus your reading on issues that matter most to you. To help you along the way, we'll explain how to use specialized lab tests and wearable technology to create a custom wellness plan designed for you.

Wearables and the science of you

There is a revolution in healthcare. We are starting to understand that one size doesn't fit all. Since we each have our own biology and respond differently, our medical care needs to be customized.

The problem is that up to now, doctors haven't had an easy way to check whether our treatment recommendations actually worked.

Imagine this. You go to the doctor to treat your high blood pressure (hypertension). Your doc prescribes you a medication, recommends that you decrease your salt intake (as they often do), and sends you on your way. You're bummed because you now have to miss out on some of your favorite foods and take a potentially toxic drug. How do we determine whether the doctor's advice is working? Beyond that, how do we know whether you even have hypertension?

Of course, you want your hypertension treated, but you don't want to use the wrong medicine and you certainly don't want to skip out on chow mein if you don't have to.

How do we know whether the doctor's treatment is right for you? The current system is to start you on a drug and then have you return to the office a couple of months later for a repeat blood pressure check. Based on this one reading, the doc will decide whether the treatment plan is working or if she needs to try something new.

Think about that for a second. One blood pressure reading, just a snapshot in time, is all the data the doctor currently has to decide whether to continue or modify a potentially life-changing medication.

How do we know that that one blood pressure reading is actually representative of anything? That one measurement could be off for countless reasons. Maybe the cuff is too small?

Were you running late to the appointment and felt nervous? Perhaps you just had an argument with your teenage daughter that morning and you're agitated. What if you just had a huge (and unhealthy) business dinner last night and drank a bit more than you should.

That one follow-up blood pressure check in the clinic can completely mislead your doctor and result in bad medical care.

That's why we need a new way to monitor how folks respond to treatment. We can't rely on generalizations or snapshot measurements. We need something better, something that shows us how someone responds over time.

Thankfully, we now have wearable technology. Small, wireless gizmos that you wear on your finger, forehead, abdomen, or wrist can measure your health. They can monitor your pulse, oxygen levels, blood pressure, and the quality of your sleep. These electronic wonders can continuously track your blood sugar and measure important labs.

In my clinics, we employ these cutting-edge devices to create customized treatment plans. We use the patient's actual (and real-time) response to food and medicine to guide medication management and dietary changes. In my view, that's the only safe way to make dietary recommendations and prescribe chronic medications. We'll cover how to use wearable technology to fight aging in chapter 4.

Who Should Read 'Why Doctors Skip Breakfast'

You wake up in the morning feeling groggy. Work is harder than it used to be. You're less focused, less energetic, and less creative. Your mood is off.

You go to your best friend and he says you're just getting older. You visit your doctor and she says that everything checks out fine. Everyone tells you to get some more sleep, exercise, and broccoli.

To make matters worse, the mirror is no longer your friend. The face staring back is losing its vitality. Your dimples transform into wrinkles and your hair grows gray. The bags under your eyes darken. Where did your youth go?

This book is designed for anyone who wants to stay young and feel happy. If you want to take charge of your future and believe that decline is not your destiny, this book is for you.

Do you grapple with any of the following:

- Decreased energy level
- Poor mood with frequent feelings of self-doubt
- Depression
- Difficulty focusing
- Loss of creativity
- Falling ambition
- Poor sleep
- Trouble waking up and getting out of bed
- Brain fog
- New lines and wrinkles
- Signs of aging—including the recent development of new chronic disease

If you struggle with any of the above, this book is your new best friend. Cutting-edge doctors already know how to maintain focus and prevent aging, and so should you.

Are you already prosperous but looking for an edge? I regularly work with top athletes, coaches, entertainers, executives, and professionals to help them reach the pinnacle of success. Exercise, practice, and good diets are important— but they aren't enough. These folks want my help to push them over the top. They want to be the best. If you are already an elite performer, read on and discover how to up your game.

I will share these breakthrough secrets with you. Why Doctors Skip Breakfast will pull back the curtain on the critical dietary tweaks, wearable gadgets, and supplements that will boost your achievement to the next level.

We keep it simple

People call me the easy-peasy guy. Although this book is written by a doctor, we won't get bogged down in excessive jargon or needless detail. I won't bore you. There will be no unnecessary talk of ribosomes, RNA, and free radicals. I'm not trying to show off. Rather, I'll explain the modern science of youth, mood, and sleep in a way that's easy to understand and use.

I've done the hard work of sifting through the research for you. There's no need for you to suffer through dry scientific papers or listen to endless podcasts. I'll cut to the chase and show you what you need to know for radiant health. Unlike many self-help books, the remarkable lifestyle interventions detailed here are based entirely on rigorous research and are explained by a master physician. For those looking to read more, there is a comprehensive reference guide at the end of Why Doctors Skip Breakfast full of recommended books and articles suitable for people of every education level.

By the time you finish reading this book, you'll know what to eat, which wearable devices to use, and what pills you need to achieve peak health and enjoy the best sleep of your life.

There's no mumbo jumbo here. Just the formula you need for success.

Definitions

Since I want you to read and use the tips in this book, I intentionally keep the writing as clear and simple as possible. The goal is for you to take action without getting bogged down in needless detail, acronyms, and esoteric concepts. Having said that, this book is based on hard science. There are a few definitions and principles that you should understand to get the most out of Why Doctors Skip Breakfast. To make life easier, I condensed most of the technical stuff into the next few pages. Feel free to read this section now or refer back as you need. I promise the rest of the book is more exciting.

Definitions and concepts:

Protein - Proteins are large, complex molecules made from amino acids. They perform a variety of important tasks throughout your body. Enzymes, antibodies, transporters, and some hormones are proteins. Proteins play an important role in maintaining structure, particularly in muscle. When you eat protein, your body breaks it down into amino acids. You'll then burn the amino acids for energy, convert them to fat or rearrange them into other proteins.

DNA - Deoxyribonucleic acid, otherwise known as DNA, is the genetic material found in nearly every cell of your body. You inherit DNA from each of your parents and you'll pass your DNA on to your offspring. Think of your DNA as your body's master database of information, as it codes for all of the genes that make you, you. Although your body is remarkably skilled at making identical copies of DNA for each of your cells, it is possible to have DNA mutations. Radiation, free radicals, and copying errors are some of the main causes of DNA mutations. Damaged DNA can trigger disease, cancer, and cellular senescence (see below).

Genes - Genes are portions of DNA and they typically code for proteins. You have two copies of most genes, one from each parent. Consider the gene for eye color. Depending on which version (or allele) of eye color genes you inherited from your mom and dad, you'll either have blue, green, or brown, etc. eyes. Humans have about 20,000-25,000 genes.

Chromosomes - Human DNA is huge. Since it's so long, it needs to be organized to prevent it from spreading out of control. A long strand of DNA is intermittently wrapped around balls of protein called histones. Imagine a super-long thread with a series of spools. The thread is the DNA and the spools are the histones. The tied-up collection of the thread and spools would be the chromosome. Humans have 46 chromosomes, 23 from each parent. Chromosomes help organize DNA, contribute to gene expression (see below), and assist in DNA duplication when a cell divides.

Telomeres - Just like the small plastic caps at the end of your shoelaces, telomeres protect the tips of chromosomes. Telomeres help preserve the structural integrity of chromosomes and defend DNA from damage. As chromosomes reproduce, telomeres can shorten. Short telomeres are a sign of cellular aging. Many of the recommendations in this book are designed to preserve or lengthen telomeres.

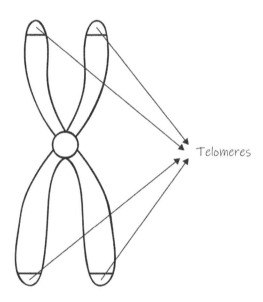

Telomeres protecting the tips of your chromosomes

Epigenetics - Consider this. You have all kinds of specialized cells in your body, like muscle cells and kidney cells. Your muscle and kidney cells are completely distinct. They make different proteins, look different under the microscope, and serve different functions. Moreover, a muscle cell cannot transform into a kidney cell and vice versa. Yet they have the same DNA. How is that possible? Let me give you another example. All of your cells with DNA have genes capable of producing every kind of protein your body can manufacture. Yet your skin cells never produce the digestive proteins assembled by your liver or pancreas. Why is that? You can thank epigenetics. Each of your cells can switch genes on and off by attaching minor, reversible tags to their DNA. These tags (methylation) can activate or silence genes, but they do not alter the underlying DNA. For example, your skin cell may attach a tag to a gene that produces a digestive enzyme to keep it turned off. Interestingly, these epigenetic tags can be passed on when cells divide and can pass from parent to offspring. Over time, there can be epigenetic errors in which the wrong genes are turned on or off. Epigenetic mistakes are believed to be a major (and reversible) causes of aging.

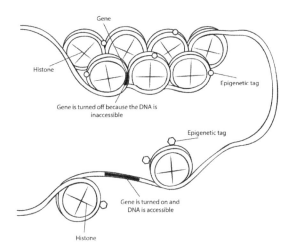

Senescent cells - Senescent cells are old or damaged cells that no longer replicate. Cellular senescence is typically caused by DNA damage or short telomeres. While everyone has some senescent cells, they're much more prevalent in the elderly. They're often called zombie cells because they don't reproduce, don't do their jobs, and just won't die. For example, a senescent liver cell sticks around and takes up space but doesn't do the work that liver cells are supposed to do. The trouble with senescent cells is that they release inflammatory cytokines (see below) in a desperate call for help. The chronic inflammatory damage caused by zombie cells is one of the major causes of aging.

Stem cells - Stem cells are undifferentiated and have the ability to transform into other cell types. While they're more common in embryos, adults have them as well. They are important for healing and they help to fight aging. Our goal is to protect your stem cells. Many of the techniques in this book will revitalize your stem cells and save them from senescence.

Apoptosis - Apoptosis is organized, programmed cell death. Think of it as cellular suicide. It is a relatively clean process whereby unnecessary or damaged cells die without harming their neighbors. As gruesome as it sounds, apoptosis is critical for health. Imagine that one of your cells suffers from DNA damage due to radiation. This mutated DNA might lead to cancer. Thankfully, that abnormal cell can fall on the sword and undergo apoptosis, nipping potential cancer in the bud. Ideally, most of our senescent cells would commit apoptosis to protect the body from their toxic shenanigans.

Inflammation - There are two types of inflammation, acute and chronic. Acute inflammation is a useful response to injury. For example, if you cut your foot, your immune cells rush to the area to fight off potential pathogens. Acute inflammation helps prevent infection. Conversely, chronic inflammation is unhelpful and maladaptive. Chronic inflammation can be caused by smoking, visceral (belly) fat, stress, unhealthy foods, lack of sleep, obstructive sleep apnea, autoimmune diseases, atherosclerosis, and toxins. Chronic inflammation is aging. The healing techniques in this book will cool down your chronic inflammation.

Cytokines - Cytokines are small proteins (peptides) that cells use to communicate with each other. While cytokines have numerous functions, for the purpose of this book, I'll be referring to the cytokines cells release to trigger inflammation. Senescent cells or cells irritated by smoking or other toxins will release cytokines that rev up the immune system and provoke an inflammatory response. Local cytokine release is one of the reasons that senescent cells cause aging.

Hormetic stress (hormesis) - It turns out that a little bit of stress is good for you. Small exposures to certain toxins will actually make you stronger and healthier. These minor stressors are healthy because they trigger you to beef up your natural defenses and repair systems. For example, when you lift weight at the gym (stress), your body responds by strengthening your muscles. Other possible hormetic stressors are radiation, free radicals, cold, difficult cognitive tasks, some bitter chemicals in spices and veggies, and fasting. Hormesis is one of your best tools in the fight against aging.

Antagonistic pleiotropy - For the purposes of aging and this book, antagonistic pleiotropy means that certain genes or proteins are helpful for younger animals before reproductive age but harmful for older animals after reproductive age. To put it another way, imagine that gene Q has two effects, one effect is helpful for teenagers and the other effect is harmful to the elderly. Natural selection might promote the spread of gene Q because it would benefit people of reproductive age. Antagonistic pleiotropy is thought to be related to senescence and appears to contribute to aging.

Glucose - A fancy medical term for a type of sugar. This book uses blood sugar and glucose interchangeably.

Mindfulness/gratitude - Your mind and body are one. To heal your body, we need to heal your mind. For the purposes of this book, I'm grouping meditation, mindfulness, gratitude, and certain exercises like yoga, tai chi, and qigong into one group—mindfulness and gratitude. While they're all different (more detail in chapter 3) they all appear to be anti-aging. They reduce stress and boost telomeres.

Microbiome - The human microbiome refers to the roughly 100 trillion microorganisms (bacteria, viruses, protozoa, and fungi) that live in or on our body, mostly in our intestines. Humans evolved with these organisms and they play a critical role in both health and disease. They support our immune system, produce some vitamins, manufacture neurotransmitters, influence our brains, and aid in digestion. A healthy and diverse microbiome protects you from aging and depression. Unfortunately, obstructive sleep apnea (OSA) sickens your gut microbes. Eat a variety of veggies and fruit to promote a healthy microbiome.

Healthspan - Lifespan is the total number of years someone is alive. By contrast, healthspan is the period of time someone is relatively free of significant illness. Imagine Janet is completely healthy until she develops high cholesterol at age 50. She continues to live a normal life until she suffers a stroke at age 86. She lives the last few years of her life in a nursing home and passes away at age 99. Her health span is 86 years and her lifespan is 99 years. For most people, the goal is to maximize healthspan.

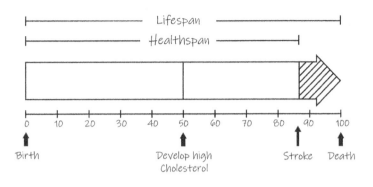

Age in Years

Ketones - Ketones are small molecules that your body (particularly your brain) can use for energy. They're produced in the liver from fat when your blood glucose and insulin run low. You can also consume ketones in supplements. While excessive ketones can be dangerous (diabetic ketoacidosis), it is believed that modest levels of ketones are beneficial for the brain. They appear to increase focus and energy. They might make you smarter by triggering the growth of new nerve cells and neuronal connections.

Diseases of aging - The most common age-associated ailments are heart disease, stroke, dementia, osteoporosis, cataracts, wrinkles, frailty, most cancers, type 2 diabetes, reduced energy, impaired cognition, sexual dysfunction, and osteoarthritis. While it's true that these diseases can impact people of all ages, they're more common and severe in the elderly. The goal of this book is to nip aging in the bud and prevent these diseases as a group.

Longevity Regulators - Your longevity regulators are genes, coenzymes, and proteins battling to keep you young and healthy. They repair DNA, fix epigenetic errors, and generate energy. The goal of this book is to marshal all of your longevity regulators to work on your behalf to protect you from the ravages of age. Examples of longevity regulators are the sirtuins, mTOR, heat shock proteins, AMPK, and NAD. For optimum health, some need to be switched on and others need to be dialed down. Hormetic stress, fasting, dietary changes, medications, and certain supplements will get your longevity regulators pointing in the right direction. Most of the recommendations in the next two chapters will focus on recruiting your longevity regulators to protect you from aging.

Phew! Now that that's done, let's get to the good stuff— how to stay young.

Chapter 2

Is Aging Preventable?

Angela has quite the competitive streak. She was the prom queen in high school and the best athlete on her Ivy League's tennis team. After graduation, she spent a year in China to visit her family and practice Mandarin. When she returned from her travels, she graduated at the top of her MBA class.

Due to her remarkable combination of beauty, brains and ambition, success came easy.

Now a young sixty, she's the CEO of a major restaurant chain based in New York. Despite her grueling work schedule, she hits the tennis courts every weekend. Angela loves life and has no plans to retire.

But her crazy schedule and endless drive hide her growing self-doubt. Tennis doesn't come as easily as it once did. She's suffering from random injuries and sprains that she never experienced before. She can't play for hours like she once did. Is she just out of practice?

While Angela still kills it in the boardroom, she loses steam once she's back in her office. She's more tired and distracted. Her laser-like focus isn't what it used to be. For the first time, she dozed off while reading the quarterly report. Is she losing a step?

To make matters worse, her doctor just told her that she has early signs of cataracts and needs to start medication for high blood pressure. Is her health in decline?

She returns home from her doctor's office shaken. Stumbling to the bathroom, she peers into the mirror. There, in the glass, she sees her elderly mom staring back at her. The wrinkles, the fatigue, the medicine cabinet full of pills. She remembers her mom's battles with osteoporosis and heart disease. After a heart attack, her mom was never the same. Now, for the first time in her life, Angela comes face to face with her own decline.

Painful memories flash before her eyes. Did Angela just see her future?

She clicks off the light and walks out to her sun-drenched patio. No, she insists. She will be the author of her own destiny. She will age the same way she's lived her whole life, on her terms.

There will be no surrender.

We are living longer

If you asked someone in 1850 how long they would expect to live, they'd shoot for the ripe old age of 40. Forty! You'd be lucky if you retired at age 39 and spent a few good years with your grandkids.

How times have changed.

Table 1. Life expectancy over time

Time period	Average human life expectancy (in years)
Classical Roman era (around 100 AD)	25
Late medieval England (around 1500)	30
England 1851	40
England 1950	68
England 2010	80

Let's look at that in a graph—just for effect:

Life Expectancy vs. Time period

As you can see, average lifespans keep increasing—and they show little sign of slowing. Lifespans improved dramatically in the 1700s and 1800s due to gains in nutrition, sanitation, infectious disease management, and child mortality. In the 1900s and early 2000s, we made great strides in treating the chronic illnesses of adults, including cancer and heart attacks.

Thankfully, it is now rare for someone to die in childbirth. In developed countries, diarrhea is an annoyance—not a death sentence. Smallpox, measles, and polio have all but vanished. An iron lung is a museum piece, not a fact of life. We've come a long way.

We're living longer, but not always healthier

As great a job as we've done in improving the duration of life, we've done a poor job of improving the quality of health in our later years. Far too many folks suffer from debilitating illnesses like chronic fatigue, brain fog, broken hips, vision loss, and shortness of breath.

We're living longer, but our bodies and brains are aging. We grow frail.

Yes, we have more years, but many of those years are spent feeling unwell. Our aged often spend the final decade of their lives in wheelchairs or nursing homes. They're unable to work. They're unable to play. And they're unable to enjoy life the way they did in their youth.

The lives of our elderly are stuffed full of doctor visits, pills, and hopelessness.

Let me give you a thought experiment. Imagine I offered you an elixir that would magically cause you to live to 110. Would you take it?

My guess is that you might say no. You'd refuse all those extra years out of fear that you'd suffer through decades of illness and dependency. You'd worry about being a burden on your family. What good is a bunch of extra years if those years are riddled with physical and mental decay?

You'd be afraid that you'd have a longer lifespan without a longer healthspan. Unfortunately, this is how we think of old age. We see the elderly as suffering from chronic illness.

But does it need to be this way?

Aging is not our destiny

We have all been told that certain things are inevitable, like death, taxes, kids turning into terrors in middle school, and aging. While there's no escaping the first three, the fourth is optional.

You read that right.

We were all told the same thing. There's a certain pathway that our lives are designed to follow. It goes something like this:

Table 2. Life expectations by age

Age	Description
Youth (birth to age 6)	Learn to walk and talk, play in the dirt, jump in muddy puddles, have fun, energy, and vitality. Eat Lego pieces off the ground.
School-age (7 to 22)	Learn to read and write. Study geometry and history. Join a rock band and dream about the future. Eat ice cream.
Adulthood (23 to 65)	Give up the rock band. Work. Buy a house. Raise a family. Two weeks of vacation per year. Care for elderly relatives. Gradual decline in energy. Insomnia and sleepless nights. Drink coffee.
Retirement years (66 - 80s)	Quit working. Take a cruise, illness, fatigue, disability, decline, nursing home. Constipation. Drink prune juice.

Are aging and frailty inevitable?

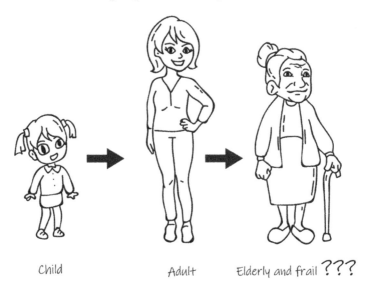

Child   Adult   Elderly and frail ???

But, is this pathway set in stone? Is it hardwired into our bodies that we have all the fun and energy in our early years and fatigue and frailty in the later ones? Do we need to suffer from heart disease, cancer, osteoporosis, Alzheimer's, and wrinkles as we age? Do we have to die before our hundredth birthday?

Top scientists and doctors say no.

It turns out that aging is no more our destiny today than tuberculosis was in the 1900s. Aging is a disease, and we can prevent it.

Sure, you'll continue to gain chronological years. There's no avoiding those. But we can prevent the maladies that we associate with aging. It turns out that most of the disabilities linked to aging share the same fundamental causes.

Heart disease, adult cancers, stroke, cataracts, saggy skin, weak bones, decreased energy levels, muscle loss, memory loss, and dementia are all tied in with aging - and all of them can be reduced or eliminated by blocking the biological pathways that cause aging. In other words, if you stop the problem at the source, you can eliminate most of the downstream effects.

Imagine that you have a nice wooden table that you leave outdoors. Over time, the sun will cause the paint to fade. Rain and moisture will cause warp. Termites will chew up the wood. Now, you could fight one of these at a time. You can put on new coats of paint, keep drying out the wood after rainstorms, and spray bug killer. Or you could just bring the table indoors and prevent all of those problems. One simple solution, bringing the table inside eliminates all of the other problems with the table.

Of course, the table still won't last forever. Nothing does. Eventually, it will break. But it will last much longer indoors than it would outside.

Think of this book as the equivalent to bringing the table indoors. You make one major change and nip your age-related problems in the bud.

The causes of aging

We used to think that aging was caused by the slow accumulation of damage to our bodies over time. With each passing year, we'd suffer little insults and irreversible DNA mutations until our body parts fail. Much like the wooden table in the example above, people felt that the body slowly decays until it collapses.

Sure, we always knew that we could do certain things to hasten or slow our decline. Smoking, radiation, and chronic stress accelerate our demise, while broccoli and exercise buy us more time. But we believed that the ravages of old age would eventually descend upon us. Sooner or later, we'll all get hit with heart disease, cancer or Alzheimer's.

Here is the big news. Science just shattered our understanding of aging. It turns out that aging isn't the gradual decay we once thought. Rather, it is caused by changes in the activity of certain genes and proteins.

This is great news. If aging were just the slow deterioration of the body over time, it would be tough to fix without literally turning back the clock. But, since aging is caused by a few troublesome genes, short telomeres and zombie cells, we can use targeted therapies and reverse the effects of age.

Thankfully, humans aren't wooden tables. We're much more complex—and resilient.

While the three primary causes of aging are distinct problems, they have overlapping causes (i.e. inflammation). Let's take a closer look at each one.

Epigenetic errors - As discussed in chapter 1, epigenetics is the reversible activation or inhibition of genes. As you age, you start turning off some beneficial genes and turning on harmful ones. Our goal here is to flip the right switches to activate your fountain of youth genes and flip off the toxic ones that are dragging you down.

Why do we have epigenetic problems? Our cells accumulate reversible errors over time. They're not dangerous enough to immediately kill the cells, but they lead to the production of harmful proteins. These harmful proteins cause age-related changes, resulting in damage to your skin, brain, and other organs. In addition, some epigenetic changes are an example of antagonistic pleiotropy, genes that are good for you when you're young (like mTOR) but aren't so great for your health when you're older.

I'll show you how to activate your longevity regulators and recruit them in your fight against these harmful errors.

Short telomeres - As your cells divide and reproduce, the telomeres (or caps that protect the end of your chromosomes) can shorten. Once telomeres get too short, the chromosomes (and cells) are unable to reproduce anymore. Let's use an example. Think of a skin cell on your cheek. Try to visualize the chromosomes in that cheek cell as a fresh pair of shoelaces. With age and injury, your skin cell keeps dividing to make up for lost cells and keep your face looking fresh. Each time the skin cell divides to make babies, the tips of the shoelaces shrink a tiny bit. Eventually, the caps are so short that the cell's chromosomes are unable to reproduce. At that point, the cell is old. It sits around, weak, frail, and possibly senescent. Imagine what happens when lots of your skin cells have short telomeres. You will look aged. This occurs throughout your body. Short telomeres, therefore, are considered a hallmark of cellular aging.

Our goal is to prevent your telomeres from shrinking. Many of the tips in the book will preserve (and possibly even lengthen) your telomeres.

Zombie cells - Senescent cells are called zombie cells because they don't die, reproduce, or do their jobs. For example, zombie skin cells don't manufacture proteins necessary to keep your skin strong and healthy. Even worse, your zombie cells release cytokines that trigger inflammatory damage to nearby cells. These buggers just stick around and cause trouble. Older people can build up critical mass senescent cells, causing dysfunction and inflammation throughout the body. The strategies in this book will reduce the production of zombie cells. We'll also fine-tune your immune system, so your body will clear away these nasty cells (immunosurveillance).

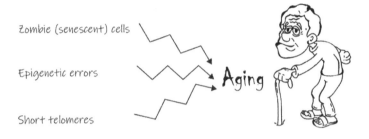

Zombie (senescent) cells

Epigenetic errors

Short telomeres

Aging

The three main causes of aging

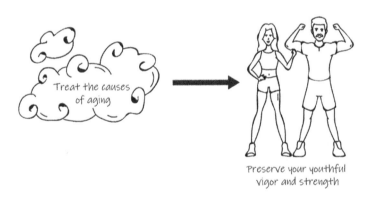

Treat the causes
of aging

Preserve your youthful
vigor and strength

Treat the causes of aging and stay young and healthy

Previous popular misconceptions about health

Let me tell you a story. Imagine that it's the mid-1800s in London. You're strolling down the cobblestone road and your foot is smashed by a horse in a sudden carriage accident. You're whisked to the hospital to repair your broken leg. It's a bad break, a compound fracture, with bone sticking out and awful pain. Darned reckless horse drivers.

The surgeon rushes in to see you. Dr. Sawhands is a delightful man in his 30s. You breathe a little easier because he's sporting scrubs caked in dried blood, the blood from all of his previous patients. You feel reassured because you know all that red residue is a sign of his experience and wisdom.

It's time for the exam. Without washing his hands, he pulls an instrument out of his pocket to probe for pus in your foot. It's dull and well-worn, having searched for milky-white pus in countless patients before you. Thankfully, you're not infected (yet).

The nurse whisks you into the operating theatre and the surgeon repairs your broken leg. The surgery is a success. Drying his freshly bloody hands on his coat, he gives you a nice slap on the back and says that he'll see you tomorrow.

You're brought upstairs to your room on the ward. The windows are open to clean out the bad air, or miasma, from the building. What a cutting edge hospital. Your sheets are a bit stiff and crunchy since they're unwashed and soiled from your bed's previous occupant. No worries, you think. At least the air is fresh. Your roommate tells you that someone passed away in your very bed last night from an infection.

After chit-chatting for a bit, you turn out the lights, pull up the covers, and settle in for the evening.

Surprisingly, you wake up the next morning to find your foot terribly infected. You call for the surgeon.

Now, as shocking and unsettling as this story is, this is how we used to deal with infections. Before Joseph Lister and his colleagues came along and proposed the germ theory of disease, people used to believe that infection was caused by bad air.

They didn't wash their hands, clean sheets, or sterilize the surgical tools because they didn't believe that tiny microorganisms living on the fluid-stained surfaces could cause infection. It was impossible to accept that something you couldn't see could be that important.

But, once we realized the true cause of infection, we were able to treat it and make hospitals much safer places. One little intervention, washing, was enough to slice maternal mortality and transform hospitals into places of healing rather than disease.

The modern science of aging is much the same. For years, we blamed aging on gradual decay. We refused to believe that a few little genes and proteins could be the cause of nearly all of the maladies of old age. But, just like Joseph Lister in the past, today's top scientists like David Sinclair, Elizabeth Blackburn, Nir Barzilai, and Leonard Guarente have unlocked the specific biological causes of aging.

Now that we understand the causes of aging, it's time to turn back the clock.

Chapter 3

How to Reverse Aging

PART I - Food

I've just told you that everything you know about aging is wrong.

Cancer, weak bones, wrinkled skin, low energy, arthritis, poor eyes, heart disease, and Alzheimer's aren't inevitable. They're preventable.

Now, I'm going to show you how.

This chapter is your how-to guide to preserve your youthful vitality. We'll go through step-by-step instructions. Everything in this chapter is easy to understand, and most steps are easy to do. No mumbo jumbo. You'll be surprised how simple it is to achieve durable, radiant health.

The tips in this chapter are based on the most cutting-edge science. The field of anti-aging research is relatively new, and exciting studies come out daily. My goal here is to bring you fresh research hot off the press that you can use right away.

Here are my (mostly) easy tips to prevent aging, improve your focus, and increase your health span:

Coffee

I'm starting this list off with my favorite. Coffee is one of the few things in life that's enjoyable and good for you. You can truly have your cake, I mean coffee, and eat it too. Let's take a look at the health benefits of coffee:

- You'll live longer. Enough said.

- It's good for your heart. Coffee decreases your risk of heart attack, stroke, and heart failure (CHF).

- It helps prevent diabetes. Your morning cup of Joe will reduce your risk of type 2 diabetes and may improve your blood sugar control.

- Alzheimer's disease. Coffee will help protect you from Alzheimer's. Drinking two or more cups a day will reduce your overall risk of dementia.

- Parkinson's disease. Coffee helps prevent Parkinson's and reduces symptoms if you already have the disease.

- Reduced risk of certain types of cancer. Coffee appears to protect you from cancer of the colon, brain, thyroid, and liver.

- Enhanced athletic performance. Leading athletic organizations including the IOC recognize caffeine as a performance enhancer. Coffee and caffeine are helpful for athletic performance when you consume them around the time of your athletic activity. Drinking coffee every morning won't help you with your late-afternoon track meets. You want to be strategic. I always discuss caffeine timing with my athlete clients. Here's why reasonable doses of coffee are so awesome for athletes:
  - Caffeine increases endurance
  - Cyclists pedal further
  - Sprinters run faster
  - Soccer stars have more speed
  - Experienced basketball players jump higher and perform better overall

- o Rugby players pass better
- o Tennis players shoot better
- o Weightlifters bench-press more
- o Coffee improves focus during workouts
- o Weightlifters have less pain after workouts

• Decreased risk of depression and suicide. Caffeinated coffee (but maybe not tea) appears to reduce the risk of depression and improves mood.

• Antioxidants. Coffee is packed with over one thousand anti-inflammatory compounds. The rich variety of antioxidants will help you ward off one of the main drivers of aging, inflammation. Coffee has so many nutrients, your cup of Joe may give blueberries a run for their money.

• Improved fasting. Coffee makes fasting (see below) easier and possibly more effective. And, black coffee won't break your fasts.

• Weight-loss. Coffee is a great appetite suppressant.

Please remember, the coffee is the healthy part, not all the junk you add to it. A Starbucks Venti Mocha Cookie Crumble Frappuccino® is loaded with 590 calories and 76 grams of sugar. I don't care how much coffee that drink contains, it isn't good for you.

The best way to drink coffee is black, either cold or iced. You can also mix in some organic cream, soy, or coconut milk. Sometimes I'll add oat milk for a treat. If you need it sweetened, try some stevia. Expresso is another tasty option.

The timing of coffee consumption is important. Don't down a watermelon-sized pitcher of coffee in the morning and then call it a day. You'll give yourself a caffeine explosion and then a crash. Rather, you want to nurse your coffee throughout the morning and early afternoon. Avoid drinking caffeine later in the afternoon as it can stick around for hours and can disrupt your sleep. Some people are slow caffeine metabolizers and need to be particularly careful about drinking coffee later in the day.

If you're an athlete, enjoy your coffee just before (or during) your event. If too much time passes between the caffeine and the competition, you'll lose the benefits. Be sure to check the rules, as some sports leagues impose restrictions on caffeine consumption.

Intermittent fasting

The light of the world will illuminate within you when you fast and purify yourself.

~Mahatma Gandhi

Fasting is the first principle of medicine; fast and see the strength of the spirit reveal itself.

~Rumi

I fast for greater physical and mental efficiency.

~Plato

I don't eat breakfast, and neither should you.

Here's why: of all the dietary changes we've tried with animals, fasting and calorie restriction are the only interventions that dramatically extend lifespan.

Sure, you can play around with keto, high-fat, low-fat, and organic diets. You can encourage the animals to exercise, adjust their light levels, add vitamins, and throw in extra fresh veggies. Those are all great. But, nothing adds to life like restricting food.

Fasting is the single most important step you can take to turn back the clock and reverse aging. At the risk of offending the cereal companies, breakfast is poison.

For millennia, philosophers, scientists, and writers have been warning us about the dangers of excessive eating. Most major world religions, including Judaism, Islam, Catholicism, Buddhism, and Hinduism hold fasting sacred. It's time we in the modern era get with the program.

In this section, we'll review the benefits of fasting, explain why fasting is so beneficial, and then explore some fasting tips and techniques. Let's start with the benefits.

Benefits of fasting:

Live longer - Quick. How do you make a monkey live to 120 person-years? Fast it. In species as diverse as mice, rats, yeast, roundworms, fruit flies, and monkeys, animals live longer when they fast. You will too. According to physician and longevity guru Dr. Peter Attia, fasting is "the single most potent tool in our toolbox of nutrition. There's nothing more potent than not eating periodically." It's much tougher to directly study the impact of fasting on lifespan in humans. A high-quality study would require randomizing some people to fast and others not to fast and then follow them over the course of their whole lives. Tough to do. Having said that, growing research in humans clearly supports the argument that fasting improves lifespan in humans.

Anti-aging - Fasting reduces the biochemical markers for aging. When you look at lab samples of fasted people, they appear to come from someone much younger. You age from the inside, and fasting reduces your biological aging.

Anti-cancer - Fasting appears to reduce the risk of several types of cancer. In animal studies, fasting even seems to slow the growth of cancer. Fasting human breast cancer survivors were less likely to have a recurrence. Even more surprising, fasting appears to boost the efficacy of chemotherapy and it reduces the incidence of chemotherapy-induced side effects.

Autoimmune diseases - Fasting improves and fine-tunes your immune system and likely decreases the risk of autoimmune diseases like multiple sclerosis, Crohn's disease, and rheumatoid arthritis.

Weight loss - Fasting is a powerful weight loss technique. In fact, some people lose so much weight fasting that they have to intentionally eat more to avoid becoming too skinny.

Healthier microbiome - It turns out that fasting isn't just good for you, it's also beneficial to the microorganisms living in your intestines. Fasting appears to increase the number of good germs while reducing the bad. The great part is that a healthier gut then creates a healthier you. Improved gut bacteria may be part of the reason fasting reduces inflammatory diseases.

Increased brainpower - I love this one. When you fast, you increase ketones, which are great brain food. You reduce the blood sugar fluctuations that kill your mood and cognitive performance. Fasting appears to enhance learning and memory. When the other doctors and I go into surgery fasted, we're focused, lucid and energized. I can tell you from personal experience, my focus is sharpest when I'm fasting. I wrote most of this book while fasting.

Hopefully, I've convinced you to start fasting. Naturally, you're probably wondering why fasting is so great. After all, we've long been taught that breakfast is the most important meal of the day.

The whole concept of the importance of breakfast came from John Harvey Kellogg and his pals in the cereal industry. Dr. Kellogg's brilliant marketing ploy still distorts our views today, over 100 years later. Let's unpack why he was wrong and review the science that explains why fasting is so beneficial. We'll need to get into a few details here because I really want you to understand why you need to make this major dietary change.

The scientific reasons why fasting is so beneficial:

Autophagy - Our bodies are full of dead weight. We're burdened with senescent and precancerous cells, misfolded proteins, and other metabolic garbage. Our goal is to rev up our immune system's capacity to identify and remove these harmful freeloaders. Think of it this way, if you were mildly staring on a desert island, your body still needs energy. What is better to burn first, your muscle or useless materials just taking up space? Evolutionarily, you're designed to burn the unnecessary stuff before going after your life-saving muscle. That's why when we challenge you with the appearance of mild food shortage, we amp up your immune system's desire to take out the cellular trash.

Longevity regulators are pushed to fight aging when we fast. These are your body's defenses against the ravages of time and we want them working on our behalf. Fasting beefs up sirtuin activity while inhibiting age-promoting mTOR.

Increased BDNF - Brain-derived neurotrophic factor (or BDNF) helps to promote the survival, growth, and function of neurons. It can even encourage the growth of new nerve cells. BDNF is important for cognitive function and memory. There is some evidence that BDNF helps to protect against Alzheimer's, stress, and depression.

Decreased IGF-1 - Reductions of insulin-like growth factor 1 (or IGF-1) may be one of the key reasons we benefit from fasting. While we need some IGF-1, lower levels appear to have an anti-aging effect. Dr. Valter Longo is one of the leading researchers in the role of IGF-1 in aging and disease, and I encourage you to follow his work.

Stem Cells - Fasting is good for stem cells. Considered one of the most promising developments in medical research, stem cells are undifferentiated cells capable of turning into almost any other cell in the body. Once a cell specializes into a liver cell, for example, it is unable to transform into a nerve, muscle, or immune cell. Since stem cells aren't yet specialized, they can turn into almost anything and heal your body. They are one of your secret weapons for regeneration. The trouble is that as we age, the number of stem cells can decline and many become senescent. Fasting increases the number of stem cells and reduces the incidence of stem cell senescence.

Hormesis - Our body does better with little stressors. The stress of lifting heavy weights, for example, encourages your muscles to grow bigger and stronger. Fasting is a form of hormesis that encourages your body to step up its game and increase resilience.

Improved mitochondrial function and energy utilization - Mitochondria are the energy factories inside our cells. It's thought that fasting boosts their efficacy and health. Fasting may also improve the ability of mitochondria to coordinate with each other and with other cellular components.

Decreased blood glucose and increased insulin sensitivity - This one is great. We'll explain this in more detail when we discuss continuous glucose monitors a little later in this chapter. Briefly, our goal is to keep your blood sugar in the low-normal range for as much of the day as possible. When we don't eat for prolonged periods, your sugar levels stay in the happy, normal range. Lower chronic blood sugar will push your insulin levels lower; low insulin levels are anti-aging and will improve your insulin sensitivity.

Good, so you're ready to try fasting (I can be pretty pushy). The question is, how should you do it? That's actually the tricky part. The best way to fast is unclear as of this writing, although we think that the longer you fast (without suffering from malnutrition), the greater the health benefits. At the end of the day, you need a program that you'll actually do. Experiment with several different fasting programs to see which works for your body and schedule.

Let's take a look at several different fasting options. Some will probably fit your lifestyle and physiology better than others. You can even combine multiple options together. Finally, we'll take a look at some tips to make your fast successful.

Fasting options:

Calorie restriction - For most people, this option is probably the most difficult. The idea with calorie restriction (CR) is that you can eat whenever you like, but you just eat less. Depending on your weight and other medical conditions, you might aim to cut around 500 calories per day. Eliminate sugary drinks, juice, and high-calorie snacks. The trouble is that many people have a hard time maintaining CR over a prolonged period. If you decide to give this one a go, you may want to contact a nutritionist for some tips. The other forms of fasting are examples of time-restricted eating.

Skip breakfast - The easiest one. Just don't eat breakfast when you wake up. Go about your day and go to school, work, or the gym. Eat lunch at lunchtime. The trick here is that you can't cheat by having a little something in the morning. If you have a banana, sugar in your coffee, or a glass of orange juice, you fell off your fast.

16:8 or 18:6 - These are 16-hour fasts followed by an eight-hour eating window or 18-hour fasts followed by a six-hour eating window. Typically these involve an early dinner and skipping breakfast. For example, if you finish dinner by 6 p.m. and your next meal is lunch at noon, you just fasted for 18 hours (18:6). Your sleep counts as part of your fast. Alternatively, if you're a big breakfast person, you can skip dinner and make lunch your last meal of the day. For example, Finish lunch at 3 p.m. and enjoy breakfast the next morning at 7 a.m. (16:8). Another term for this is time-restricted eating.

OMAD - This cool acronym stands for one meal a day. In this fasting model, you have one huge meal instead of several smaller ones. For example, you just drink water and coffee throughout the day and sit down with your family for a giant dinner. I've tried this fasting style and it's not as bad as it sounds. It can be fun to have a huge meal. In my opinion, the trouble with OMAD is it can be tough to get your whole day's supply of fruits and veggies in one meal.

5:2 - This one is a little different. For five days, you can eat whenever you like. The other two days are calorie-restricted. You just have 500-600 calories on the restricted days. For example, you eat as usual from Monday-Friday. But, you only eat around 500 calories (a smallish meal) on

Saturday and Sunday. A study of 100 overweight women in the UK showed that people on the 5:2 diet lost weight, improved their insulin sensitivity, and reduced their body fat.

Periodic prolonged fasts - Go ahead and eat whenever you want most of the time but every so often you have a long fast of 24, 36, or even 48 hours. If this is your sole form of fasting, you probably want one of these long fasts once a week or once a month. If you're combining this with another type of fasting, I recommend doing these long fasts 1-4 times per year.

In case you're curious, I use the 16:8 or 18:6 model. Now that I've done this for a while, I find it easy to do and I rarely get hungry during my fasting periods. Honestly, I feel better and think more clearly while I'm fasting. I also throw in a few longer (36 hour+) fasts every so often.

Here are some tips to make fasting easier and more effective:

Liberally drink water during your fasts - The goal is to cut out stuff with calories, not to become dehydrated.

Avoid malnutrition - Regardless of how you fast, you still need to satisfy your body's minimum nutrient requirements. You must consume all your required vitamins, minerals, essential amino acids (protein), fiber, and fatty acids. You need enough calories to meet your metabolic needs, and you still have to consume your healthy veggies. If you have any concern that you're not meeting your minimum nutritional requirements, speak with your doctor or nutritionist for advice. We want to make you healthy, not sick.

Drink black coffee and tea during your fasts - They'll give you more energy, suppress your appetite, and might even improve the quality of your fasts. There is some evidence that they'll even increase your ketones. If fasting makes you cranky and irritable, tea and coffee may take the edge off.

It gets easier - The first few days you fast can be tough. Just like with running a race, you need to train and practice. With time, your body will adapt (which was one of the main goals of fasting). Your cells will learn how to use alternative energy sources and will be more efficient. Don't give up just because the first few days were hard.

Speak to your doctor, particularly if you have any medical conditions - You'll want their advice about the safest way to fast.

You might lose weight unintentionally - While this may be a bonus for most folks, thin people will need to pay attention to their weight. Here's the deal. If you shrink your eating time per day from 16 hours to eight hours, you will naturally eat less in those eight hours than you would have in 16. If you don't want to lose weight, you may have to intentionally eat more during your limited eating window.

Experiment with different fasting strategies and times - Skipping breakfast is easy with my lifestyle. It may be different for you. Perhaps it's important for you to have breakfast with your family or work colleagues. If so, no worries. Have breakfast with them and use a different strategy like 5:2, skipping dinner, or occasional prolonged fasts.

Occasional cheating is okay - My family and I have what we call our "Saturday Morning Tradition." Nearly every Saturday morning, we go out for breakfast together. We pick a new restaurant and bring books, activities, and games. I often eat earlier (and unhealthier) than I do the other six days of the week. Fasting isn't worth giving up this important time with my family. Don't worry if you miss some of your fasts here and there.

Find other people to fast with - It's easier when you have friends who share your goals. It can be tough to fast if your crowd heads out to McDonald's every morning while you're left behind. Find a fasting buddy and go out together for a morning jog, yoga class, or trip to that new coffee shop downtown.

Elite athletes may want to be cautious about fasting. In some respects, the goal of building massive amounts of muscle can run counter to the anti-aging goals of increasing autophagy. For example, if your goal is longevity, you want to inhibit mTOR. Professional athletes want to stimulate mTOR to bulk up and gain more muscle. In addition, professional athletes need to eat A LOT of calories to compensate for their intense training sessions. It can be tough to eat enough calories if you're only eating for 6-8 hours per day. If you're a professional athlete considering fasting, I strongly advise you to consult with your training staff first.

What about recreational athletes? Should they fast? Yes! Fasting is a no-brainer for recreational athletes. You're exercising to be healthy, after all. Many people think that fasting can improve the performance, focus, and mental acuity of recreational athletes. The exercise may even boost your ketone production. I'm often asked how to time exercise with fasting. If your schedule allows, I suggest you have only coffee for breakfast, go to the gym in the late morning, and enjoy a nice lunch after. Alternatively, you can work out in the early evening after lunch and before dinner.

Consider drinking ketone esters. Ketone esters raise your ketones levels well above what you'd expect from a 16:8 or 18:6 fast. Your brain, particularly your thinking frontal lobe, fests on ketones for fuel. Ketone esters supercharge your focus and cognitive performance. They seem to be neuronal protective (anti-aging). Exogenous ketone esters might make you smarter by increasing the brain-boosting BDNF (brain-derived neurotrophic factor). Finally, athletes appear to benefit from taking exogenous ketones near their workouts.

Finally, I encourage you to make fasting fun. It can get boring consuming the same stuff each time you fast. I'm a big fan of flavored sparkling water like LaCroix, San Pellegrino, and Bubly. They come in all sorts of flavors and have no sugar or calories. I always keep a few cases in the fridge. You can also spice things up by trying different herbal teas, sampling different brands of coffee, and exploring different methods to prepare coffee (iced, cold brew, French Press, etc.).

Let me leave you with this gem:

To lengthen thy life, lessen thy meals.

~Benjamin Franklin

Continuous Glucose Monitoring

Thanks to modern technology, you now have a secret weapon in the fight against aging. I like to call it personalized wellness.

As we discussed throughout this book, high blood sugar levels are harmful to your health. Elevated blood sugar increases insulin and suppresses our beneficial longevity regulators. Our goal, therefore, is to maintain your blood sugar at the low end of the normal range (70-90 mg/dl) for as much of the day as possible. In other words, we want to keep your day's average blood sugar in the healthy sweet spot (if you'll pardon the pun).

In addition, we want to minimize spikes in blood glucose that come from eating sugary foods. These blood sugar spikes cause a corresponding insulin surge and collapse which does a number on your health, appetite, and energy level.

The trouble is, everyone is different. The way your body reacts to any particular food is different from how my body reacts.

Until now, the best advice we could give was to practice intermittent fasting, restrict calories, avoid sugary foods, and eat lots of healthy, fiber-rich veggies. And while these tips are good for the population on average, how do we know what's best for you?

Each of us reacts to foods differently, and generic eating guidelines don't capture our individual responses. Therefore, traditional dietary advice may be great for some people but horrible for others.

Let me give you an example.

You and I decide to grab lunch. We go out for sashimi and we both enjoy a nice bowl of rice with our meal. Here's the deal. Unbeknownst to us, the rice socks you with a massive surge in blood glucose, while my blood sugar barely budges.

The next day, I treat you to lunch. We both scarf down a heaping serving of potatoes (our restaurant is famous for their spuds). This time, however, you devour the potatoes without any significant effect on your blood sugar. Mine, unfortunately, shoots through the roof.

But, since neither of us knew about our body's idiosyncratic reaction to food, we didn't realize that we were needlessly poisoning ourselves day after day with unhealthy meals. If only we knew how our bodies reacted to particular foods, we could eat smarter. You could safely enjoy your fill of potatoes with your meals while I go for the rice.

Another example. Some foods, like fruit, can be a wolf in sheep's clothing. What if you knew that grapes cause your blood glucose to skyrocket while strawberries and apples are harmless? With this data, you could score free health points by skipping the grapes in your fruit salad and substituting them with a crunchy Honeycrisp.

If we knew how your body responds to any individual food, we could make personalized nutrition recommendations tailored to your body. You could fine-tune your diet to eat the meals that are right for you. In our examples, you'd eat strawberries and potatoes while skipping the grapes and rice.

Thanks to technology, this personalization is now possible.

A device called a continuous glucose monitor (CGM) measures your blood sugar level from moment to moment. With each meal and after every snack you can observe how your body reacts to food. Originally created for diabetics, this device is the perfect tool for all who seek wellness. Think of it as a window into the inner workings of your metabolism. You can buy a monitor from companies like Dexcom or Medtronic.

Here's how it works. Your physician or wellness expert places a tiny wire electrode under your skin. This electrode communicates with a small box you wear or carry nearby. Through the wonder of modern technology, the electrode is able to accurately measure your blood sugar level in almost real-time. It shares the data with your smartphone and your doctor for analysis.

Imagine it's Tuesday morning. You wake up and glance at your phone. Glucose of 83. Not bad. Your healthy early dinner last night left you in good shape. You get dressed and rush off to work. Your startup is about to release its first product and you want everything to be perfect for launch.

You break your fast early today, figuring that you should have some food in your stomach before your pre-launch meetings. You pick up a banana and granola bar from a shop on Market Street. You check your glucose during your first meeting. 170. Yikes! That early-morning snack did a number on your blood sugar.

An hour later, you start to feel sluggish. You're losing focus. One Keynote slide blends into the next. Why? You glance at your phone and see your blood glucose is only 65. Now, you have your answer.

The problem wasn't the slides, it was your snack.

After you wolfed down your seemingly harmless sweet treat, you had an explosive blood sugar response. For a while, your sugar went way too high. Your body naturally reacted by releasing a burst of insulin in an attempt to bring your glucose back down to a normal level. Unfortunately, this insulin surge went too far and your blood sugar came crashing down (hypoglycemia). This sugary roller coaster and subsequent crash are what caused your sleepiness and lack of focus during the meeting. To make matters worse, your post-snack bout of hypoglycemia makes you hungry for even more sugar. We discuss this phenomenon in more detail below.

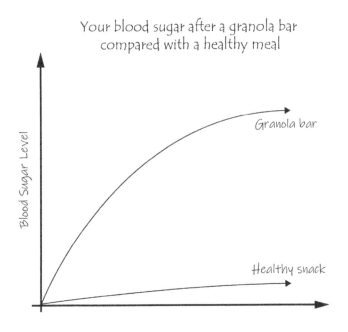

Your blood sugar after a granola bar compared with a healthy meal

Now, let's do it a better way. Your best bet would have been to skip the granola bar and instead enjoy an invigorating glass of water and some freshly-brewed coffee.

But, if you need a snack, wouldn't it be better to eat food that you know won't trigger your body to have a massive glucose spike? Imagine if you knew that oranges (as an example) have a minimal impact on your blood sugar. After all, you ate them before and watched your body's modest reaction on your continuous glucose monitor. Your research on yourself told you that oranges are a safe snack.

So, this time you grabbed an orange (and coffee) on the way to your meeting. No wild ride for your blood glucose. Now, you won't have the surge of blood sugar and there's no crash. You're awake and attentive. You feel good. And your product launch is a huge success.

#####

I recommend you speak with your medical professional or wellness doctor about using a continuous glucose monitor. If you don't have diabetes, this is an off-label use. So, your insurance won't cover it and you will likely have to pay cash, but it is well worth it.

You can either use it all the time or just try it for a week or two. The goal is to learn how your body reacts to as many different foods and fasting regimens as possible.

You may be surprised that some foods you considered "safe" will make your glucose go haywire. Perhaps you regularly indulge in a fruit and yogurt parfait at the coffee shop near work for lunch. Yogurt is healthy, after all. But now, you're armed with a tool to gather information. So, when you go this afternoon for your "healthy" lunch, you learn the parfait's dark secret. It drives your blood sugar through the roof.

[Author's note: In the above example, I'm not suggesting that you should never enjoy the parfait. Life would be dull if you're constantly denying yourself your favorite foods. Rather, I'm making the case that you shouldn't eat the parfait regularly for lunch. Understand it for what it is—it's a desert, not a meal. Go ahead and have it from time to time the way you'd have any desert. And find something else to eat for lunch.]

To get the most out of your glucose monitor, you'll want to combine it with a food diary. There are lots of great apps for this. The idea is to track what you eat and when. Then you can compare your blood sugar responses to your different meals. The technology on the glucose monitor makes it easy to review your trends throughout the day.

The monitor and diary empower you and your wellness physician to examine how the content and timing of your meals impact your body. For example, based on your sleep times and your body's natural production of the hormone cortisol, your ideal meal plan may be a large lunch at 11, a snack at 2, and dinner at 6 (notice the compressed eating window to facilitate intermittent fasting).

Why should you care about how your blood glucose responds to food? As we discussed, improved blood sugar control will boost your energy level, increase your insulin sensitivity, prevent weight gain, and reverse aging.

When your blood sugar is high, the sugar molecules will stick to your proteins and fats and create a sticky toxin called advanced glycation end-products (AGEs). AGEs will trigger inflammation, increase your risk for Alzheimer's, and quite literally cause you to age. In a sense, your high blood sugar is caramelizing your body from the inside. Yuck.

Blood glucose and energy level - As we mentioned above, wild fluctuations of blood sugar are mood and energy killers. If you eat a candy bar, your glucose will skyrocket as you absorb all that sugar into your bloodstream. This elevated glucose level will trigger your pancreas to release insulin. A lot of insulin. This insulin surge will then suck the toxic sugar out of your blood and into your cells. In particular, your fat cells (adipose tissue) are ready to feast on your sugar bolus.

The trouble is that your poor pancreas doesn't know when your sugary meal is coming to an end. So, it pumps out as much insulin as possible. Therefore, your candy bar's massive insulin spike will likely overshoot the target. Rather than just reduce your glucose to a normal level, you'll temporarily suffer low blood sugar (hypoglycemia).

Your blood sugar rollercoaster after you eat a candybar

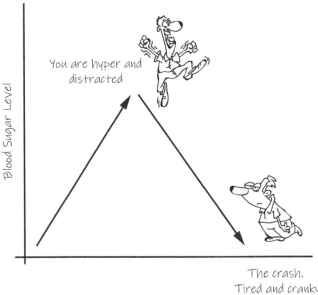

You are hyper and distracted

The crash.
Tired and cranky

Your blood sugar's wild ride is responsible for your mood and energy instability after you eat an unhealthy meal. If you have kids, you know all about this. Give little Johnny some desert and he starts bouncing off the walls. He's wild with giddy energy. But it won't last. Before long, like Dr. Jekyll and Mr. Hyde, Johnny transforms into a cranky monster. The crying, complaining, and tantrums are sure to follow. Before long, he's collapsing on the floor in the middle of Target.

Unfortunately, your body does the same thing. While you may not start crying in the toilet paper aisle, you suffer through the volatility caused by your rising and falling blood sugar. First, you're anxious and distracted. Then, you're drowsy and unfocused.

Once you understand how different foods alter your delicate body chemistry, we can put that knowledge to work for your benefit. Cut out or minimize the foods that spike your blood sugar and feast on the meals that work well for you.

What works for other people may not work for you. The continuous blood sugar monitor is your ticket for truly personalized medicine.

PART II

Supplements, medications, and labs

Metformin

Aging research reminds us that we aren't just a collection of different organs. We're one unified whole, and our body succeeds or fails as a package deal.

One "recent" discovery is the pill metformin. Developed sixty years ago as a diabetes drug, metformin might be one of the most powerful anti-aging medications available. I put "recent" in quotes because we're only just now starting to understand metformin's powerful effects on longevity. Despite what you may hear on skin cream commercials, metformin is the closest thing to the fountain of youth that you can buy today.

In organisms as diverse as roundworms, mice, rats, silkworms, and humans, metformin shows incredible promise at preventing the consequences of aging.

Metformin appears to give us longer lives and improved overall health. It helps with weight loss, diabetes management, and improved insulin responsiveness. Beyond diabetes care, metformin appears to help prevent Alzheimer's and cognitive decline, cancer, heart disease, and frailty. It even seems to relieve depression.

We don't completely understand how metformin works to improve our health. Some theorize that it works by mimicking the beneficial effects of calorie restriction in the energy-producing factories of your cells, the mitochondria.

Metformin appears to energize the anti-aging proteins AMPK and SIRT1. These remarkable longevity regulators are part of your body's defenses against the ravages of time.

Exciting new research on the importance of AMPK, SIRT1, and other longevity genes and proteins seems to come out every day.

Even better, metformin is inexpensive and relatively free of side effects. The most concerning is a serious condition called lactic acidosis. Fortunately, lactic acidosis is extremely rare. Since pre-existing kidney disease appears to increase the risk for lactic acidosis, metformin should be used with caution by people with kidney dysfunction.

Given metformin's overall safety profile and its potential to prevent diseases like cancer and dementia, I would encourage you to discuss potential metformin therapy with your doctor or anti-aging specialist. Typical doses are 850-1000 mg daily or several times a week.

Resveratrol and pterostilbene

We've all heard about the health benefits of red wine. Seniors the world over credit their longevity to their daily glass. Well, it turns out that there may be some truth to the value of red wine, and particularly the most active component, resveratrol.

Resveratrol is produced by grapes and some other plants in times of stress (like drought). It is thought that resveratrol helps the plants, along with the animals that eat them, cope with adversity (hormetic stress).

Like metformin and rapamycin (another powerful anti-aging medication), resveratrol appears to have multiple anti-aging and disease-fighting properties across the animal world. Resveratrol simply makes animals live longer. Creatures as diverse as yeast, mice, fruit flies, roundworms, and humans all benefit from resveratrol's good graces.

Beyond living longer, resveratrol is your partner in the battle against aging and disease. This miraculous molecule appears to fight heart disease, cancer, inflammation, saggy skin, and neurologic decay.

The trouble with resveratrol is that it is tough to get it in your blood. The scientific term for this is poor bioavailability. A part of the problem may be that your liver rapidly metabolizes and inactivates resveratrol and your kidneys are quick to excrete it. Sheesh, talk about looking a gift horse in the mouth. If you can't get and keep the stuff in your body, it won't do you much good.

Researchers are actively seeking the optimal way to consume resveratrol. Some data suggest that black pepper (piperine) may enhance resveratrol bioavailability. Stay tuned, as this is a fast-moving field. If you choose to take resveratrol, shoot for around 1000 mg per day.

Thankfully, there is an alternative to resveratrol that is more bioavailable. Found in the skin of blueberries and grapes, pterostilbene is in the same chemical family as resveratrol and seems to have many of the same benefits.

Pterostilbene appears to fight aging, cancer, and heart disease. Some evidence suggests that pterostilbene is superior to resveratrol for the prevention of brain dysfunction.

While there are fewer scientific studies about pterostilbene than its chemical cousin resveratrol, pterostilbene's superior potency and bioavailability probably make it a better choice as a supplement. I recommend taking 150 mg of pterostilbene per day. Alternatively, you can take both pterostilbene and resveratrol. If you'd like to take both, start with one and see how you feel. Then add the second and see how your body reacts. Since these supplements appear to have few side effects (there are some reports of GI upset), it should be easy to take both.

Finally, there is some thought that resveratrol and pterostilbene are particularly beneficial when combined with fasting. If you're practicing intermittent fasting, I strongly encourage you to add at least one of these disease-fighting superheroes (along with pepper) to your daily regimen.

NMN and NR

It's no secret that most people seem to lose energy as they age. Older folks often feel that they don't have the same pep they enjoyed in their younger years. While there are a number of causes for this decline in energy, one explanation may be the loss of a key energy-producing molecule in our cells as we age. NAD (also called NAD+ or NADH) is a component of cellular respiration and is used throughout our bodies (in conjunction with NADH) to help power nearly everything we do.

Since NAD levels fall with age, many scientists believe that the loss of NAD is partly responsible for your decline in energy, stamina, and drive as we grow older.

Beyond providing the energy for life, here are some additional critical functions of NAD:

• Maintains proper immune function

• Repairs damaged DNA

• Cellular communication

• Development and maintenance of skeletal muscle

Perhaps most importantly for this book, NAD appears to play a role in aging. In other words, when people age their NAD level falls. But, when NAD levels fall, aging is promoted. It is a vicious cycle.

Based largely on cutting-edge animal research, we now believe that boosting NAD levels will fight disease and prevent some of the ravages of aging. When you enhance an animal's NAD levels, their exercise performance skyrockets. A little NAD turns an ordinary mouse into an elite athlete. NAD improves strength, balance, and memory. It even seems to combat diabetes.

NAD appears to protect cells from oxidative stress. There is hope that NAD will protect us against heart disease, glaucoma, and Alzheimer's.

Researchers believe that NAD battles aging in humans and other animals by activating our natural longevity system, the sirtuins. NAD appears to be better than resveratrol at turbocharging our natural sirtuin survival circuits.

How do you increase your NAD levels? You can take either nicotinamide riboside (NR) or nicotinamide mononucleotide (NMN). Pop either one of those and your body's NAD concentration, energy level, and sirtuin activity will get a jolt.

Given NAD's support of sirtuins and overwhelming benefit to animals, I recommend that you try to boost your own NAD levels. NMN appears to be more stable but quite a bit more expensive than NR. As of this writing, one cannot definitively say whether you should take NR or NMN. Your goal should be 250-1000 mg of NMN or around 300 mg of NR each morning. You may want to pair NR with pterostilbene. A recent study suggested that NR may be safe up to 1000 mg per day or more.

Note: while many thought-leaders in aging research recommend using a NAD booster, the research in humans is still in its infancy. As a useful counterpoint, I included a Scientific American article in the references that discusses whether NAD boosters might prevent or promote cancer.

Unfortunately, anything that improves the health and longevity of normal cells has the potential to enhance the longevity of cancer cells. That's why it's important to work with a knowledgeable wellness physician. Based on the powerful evidence that NAD boosters increase the overall healthspan in animals, I am confident that they'll help humans as well. Visit my website for all the latest info.

Enjoy your flavors and spices: oregano, turmeric, garlic, mustard, and dark chocolate

Besides drinking more coffee, adding healthful spices and herbs may be one of the easiest and most delicious things you can do for your wellbeing. Most herbs and spices are healthy, and you should strive to include as many of them as possible in your cooking. The reason they're so good for you is that they're packed with unique phytochemicals and antioxidants that you won't find anywhere else. These health-promoting natural substances are responsible for both the flavor and color of your herbs. In fact, the same plant-derived substances that make herbs so tasty also make them healthy. Flavonoids, terpenes, and polyphenols can fight cancer, heart disease, and aging.

Here are some specific herbs that I recommend that you add to your diet. However, this list is NOT meant to be all-inclusive. You should enjoy as many delicious herbs and spices as possible. Go out to the store and experiment. It's easy and fun to add these nutritional powerhouses to your meals.

Some of my recommended herbs:

Oregano - One of nature's wonder-foods, oregano is loved the world over. It is rich in antioxidants, decreases inflammation, fights cancer, and helps prevent infections. It may be beneficial for asthma, rheumatoid arthritis, and high cholesterol. Oregano might help protect you from the harmful effects of radiation. While oregano oil is available as a supplement, I recommend liberally sprinkling the real stuff on your food. I particularly enjoy it on baked veggies, salad, pizza, and fish. It's surprising how much you can use and it always seems to taste good.

Turmeric - Responsible for the brilliant color found in many curries, turmeric is one of the healthiest foods around. Turmeric's rich, dark color is a sign of its disease-fighting prowess. Curcumin is believed to be the main active ingredient in turmeric. Turmeric has been used successfully in Asia for thousands of years for cooking and medicine. This spice has stood the test of time because it works. Research suggests that turmeric fights ulcerative colitis, depression, arthritis, heart disease, hay fever, and elevated cholesterol. It may decrease your risk of cancer, dementia, gingivitis, and inflammation. As an anesthesiologist, I'm excited to share that turmeric might even help people recover after surgery. You can add turmeric to your food and take it (curcumin) in capsules. To maximize the turmeric's bioavailability, be sure to enjoy it with black pepper. While the dose isn't clear, I recommend 1000-2000 mg per day.

Garlic - Yum! One of my favorite foods, garlic is also one of the healthiest. It's great for your cardiovascular system. It will lead the charge against heart disease, stroke, atherosclerosis, and high blood pressure. Garlic enhances the overall health of your blood vessels. This powerful herb may help prevent the common cold and Alzheimer's disease. Garlic might even improve athletic performance, although more studies are needed. I love garlic with veggies, fish, pizza, pasta (quinoa or legume pasta), and lentils. Honestly, I add garlic to almost everything I cook. Shoot for at least 800 mg (¼ teaspoon) of garlic powder or at least one clove of garlic per day. I love the Dorot frozen crushed garlic cubes from Trader Joe's. They taste fantastic and are easy to use. Note: garlic appears to offer some protection from respiratory viruses similar to COVID-19. If you're looking for natural food that might offer some benefit for COVID-19 in addition to other precautions like distance and frequent hand washing, consider increasing your intake of garlic.

Mustard - Ah, now we're on to your secret weapon. We all know that broccoli and other cruciferous veggies like cauliflower, kale, cabbage, bok choy, and Brussels sprouts are some of the healthiest foods around. A major reason why they're so healthy is they give us the superhero molecule sulforaphane. Don't let the silly name fool you, sulforaphane is good stuff. It prevents cancer better than almost anything else you can eat. It seems particularly useful in combating breast and prostate cancers. Sulforaphane helps your heart, combats diabetes, protects you from the sun, and may even help treat autism. Sulforaphane is anti-inflammatory and promotes all-important autophagy, where your body kills the nasty old cells that are hanging around and making you sick. Therefore, sulforaphane is anti-aging.

Here's the trouble. When you cook your broccoli and other cruciferous veggies, you don't get the sulforaphane. Bad news! So, here's where mustard comes in. When you add mustard powder to your cooked veggies, you bring the sulforaphane content back to normal. Mustard is Robin to sulforaphane's Batman. The mustard negates the harmful effect of cooking your broccoli. So, here's the tip. Whenever you enjoy cooked cruciferous veggies (which should be often), be sure to sprinkle some mustard powder on them before eating. It tastes great, fights aging, and will improve your health.

Dark chocolate - I know it's not really a spice. But it makes sense to discuss the health benefits of dark chocolate here. Studies suggest that this delicacy improves brain function, reduces skin damage from the sun's UV radiation, and may reduce your risk of heart disease. Packed with flavonoids and polyphenols, dark chocolate is anti-inflammatory and anti-aging. The key is that you want to eat dark chocolate that is NOT processed with alkali. Unfortunately, that form of processing reduces the health benefits of the chocolate. You also want your chocolate to be at least 70% cocoa. And, needless to say, you don't want it with a bunch of added sugar. My preference is organic fair-trade dark chocolate powder. I add it to smoothies, yogurt, oatmeal, coffee, and organic milk (from pasture-raised cows or vegan oat/flax milk). If you have a craving for dessert, have a few squares of a 70+% dark chocolate bar produced with minimal sugar.

Fish and fish oil

Omega-3s and fish oil are all the rage. You can't go into a gym, dinner party, or hair salon without someone telling you to pop some fish pills. But is it true? Are omega-3s and fish products as good as everyone claims?

First, a tiny bit of background. Because I want this book to be actionable, I've tried to not get bogged down with too many technical terms. However, I think a brief explanation of fat is in order here.

Fatty acids, the long, complex molecules that make up "fat," are ubiquitous in nature. All living things require various types of fatty acids to survive. Animals use fat to maintain cellular structure, store and transport energy, produce hormones, and to aid in the absorption and metabolism of nutrients. In short, fat is essential for survival.

Fatty acids, which are the building blocks of fat (or oil), come in three main varieties: saturated, monounsaturated, and polyunsaturated. Polyunsaturated fats can be further divided into omega-3, omega-6, and omega-9s.

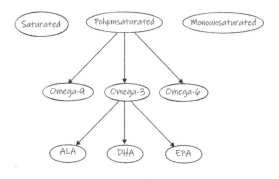

Some types of fat

67

To make matters more complicated, there are several different types of omega-3 fats. The most commonly discussed are ALA, EPA, and DHA. While all are critical for good health, it is believed that EPA and DHA are the most important. Your body can manufacture some fatty acids from scratch, but you're unable to create omega-3s de novo. In other words, omega-3 fats are essential—you need to eat some in your diet. Your body is able to convert a small amount of ALA into EPA and DHA.

To summarize, you need to consume at least some ALA, EPA, and DHA to live.

Here are common dietary sources of omega-3s:

Table 1. Sources of omega-3 fats

Type of omega-3 fat	Dietary sources
ALA (alpha-linolenic acid)	Walnuts, chia seeds, flax seeds, some grass-fed meats, Brussels sprouts, leafy green veggies
DHA (docosahexaenoic acid) and EPA (eicosapentaenoic acid)	Fatty fish (salmon, mackerel, tuna, herring, sardines, and anchovies), algae (algal oils are the best vegan source of DHA and EPA), seaweed

All right, so now that you know what omega-3 fats are and how to naturally include them in your diet, should you supplement them?

The answer appears to be yes. Here are some of the benefits of adding omega-3 fats to your diet (particularly EPA and DHA which come from fish or algae):

- Lower risk of sudden cardiac death

- Decreased risk of stroke and repeat heart attack

- Improved fetal brain development (pregnant women should speak with their obstetricians about nutrition and all supplements)

- Lower risk of depression and anxiety

- Decreased risk of macular degeneration, one of the leading causes of vision loss in the elderly

- They're anti-aging since they decrease chronic inflammation

- Improved blood pressure, heart rhythm, and blood vessel health

- They may help fight autoimmune diseases like Crohn's disease, lupus, rheumatoid arthritis, and type 1 diabetes

- Decreased risk of colon cancer

- Improved endurance and muscle recovery for elite athletes (but not increased muscle growth)

- Lower risk of Alzheimer's disease and improved overall brain health

How much omega-3 should you consume? I recommend starting first with natural foods. For ALA, snack on walnuts, add chia or ground flax seeds to your oatmeal or yogurt, and eat green leafy veggies. If you eat meat, try to purchase only organic, grass-fed animals since they have higher levels of omega-3s (and they're probably treated better).

For EPA and DHA (which is more important than ALA), you should try to eat oily fish at least three times a week. Be sure to throw a pack of seaweed in your bag and sprinkle it liberally on your salad, quinoa, and brown rice.

As for supplements, you probably want at least 500 mg of EPA combined with DHA. Some authorities recommend significantly higher doses. Vegans can substitute algal oil for fish oil. Nordic Naturals makes a great algal oil supplement.

Finally, avoid trans fats. They increase your risk of diabetes, heart disease, and stroke. They also increase your bad cholesterol level (LDL) while damaging your good cholesterol (HDL). In my opinion, the only safe dose of trans fats is zero.

Check your labs

When you get your annual physical, your doctor will check routine labs. That's not what we're talking about here. Your health goal isn't the bare minimum, you want to achieve peak physical and mental fitness.

With these tests, we'll be able to fine-tune your diet and supplement regimen to help you reach optimum performance. We'll also check to see if you're at risk for Alzheimer's disease and hidden food sensitivities.

You can't just walk into a lab (in the United States) and request these blood tests for yourself. Rather, you should ask your doctor or wellness physician to draw these labs. Some primary care providers may not be accustomed to all of these exams, so you may need to speak with a specialist for help interpreting the results.

Fasting insulin level - Part of the reason for fasting is to keep your baseline blood sugar (glucose levels) low. Your body should reward your healthy blood sugar levels by keeping your insulin levels low. Insulin, after all, is the hormone your body releases to vacuum the extra sugar out of your blood and into your cells. Low fasting insulin levels are correlated with good health and high insulin sensitivity. With low fasting insulin levels, you're less likely to develop type 2 diabetes and Alzheimer's. Shoot for an insulin level below 4.5 uIU/mL, although a level below 2 is probably best.

Hemoglobin A1c - This test measures how much glucose is stuck to your blood's hemoglobin. It's a rough approximation of your blood sugar level over time. While this test is often ordered for diabetics to track disease progress, it is useful for everyone. It will help tell you if your blood sugar is chronically high even if you don't have diabetes. Your goal here is an HbA1c level of 5.5 % or below.

Fasting blood sugar (glucose) - We want to keep this in the low-normal range. Obviously, extremely low blood sugars are dangerous and potentially fatal. People with type 1 diabetes must constantly be on guard against hypoglycemia. I am not advocating hypoglycemia. Rather, we want your blood sugar at the lower end of the normal range. Our goal is a fasting glucose of 70-90 mg/dl. In addition to the lab fasting glucose, I strongly recommend you use a continuous glucose monitor (see above).

Testosterone level (for men) - Testosterone replacement therapy has been all over the news lately. While testosterone replacement is unlikely to increase the length of life, it may improve the quality of life. Suspected benefits of testosterone replacement include improved mood, self-confidence, increased strength, reduction in osteoporosis, and enhanced sex drive and performance. It appears likely that testosterone replacement also improves focus and cognitive performance in some men. There is also some research that suggests that testosterone replacement reduces the risk of Alzheimer's disease. Your goal total testosterone level should be 500-1000 ng/dL (probably closer to 1000) and a free testosterone level of 6.5-15 ng/dL.

Homocysteine - Homocysteine is a byproduct of amino acid (protein) metabolism. When you eat large amounts of foods high in the amino acid methionine, like beef, turkey, fish, pork, eggs, and nuts, you may increase your homocysteine levels. You then convert the homocysteine into harmless substances using vitamin B12 and other B vitamins. Some people are also genetically prone to elevated homocysteine levels. High levels of homocysteine can increase your risk of heart disease and Alzheimer's disease. Your goal homocysteine level is 6 μmol/L or less.

ApoE4 - This test is optional and has some ethical implications, but you should consider it if you're concerned about your risk for Alzheimer's disease. The ApoE4 gene is considered the strongest genetic risk factor for the development of Alzheimer's disease. Here's the deal. You inherit one copy of the APOE gene from your mother and one from your father. Thus, each of us has two copies of the gene. The APOE gene has three flavors, ApoE2, ApoE3, and ApoE4. Therefore, depending on what you inherited from each of your parents, you can have any mixed pair combo of the three different types of APOE genes. Think of it the same way you might inherit a gene for eye color from your parents. Perhaps you got a brown-eye gene from your mom and a blue-eye gene from your dad. You could have ApoE2/ApoE2, ApoE2/ApoE3, ApoE4/ApoE3, and so on.

The reason this is important is that if you have a copy of the ApoE4 gene, you're more likely to develop Alzheimer's than someone who doesn't have it. If you have two copies, you have an even greater risk. If you want to better understand your future risk for Alzheimer's disease, you might want to get this gene tested.

Before you get the test, you should consider the ethical implications. The first consideration is deciding whether you want to know your risk of developing a serious disease in the future that you have only limited ability to prevent. The second consideration is that you're not only finding out your risk, you're also learning about the risk of your parents, siblings, and kids. For example, if you're ApoE4/ApoE4, you know that your parents each must have at least one copy of the ApoE4 gene. In this example, each of your kids will also have at least one copy of the ApoE4 gene (from you).

Finally, I want to say that having the ApoE4 gene is not a guarantee you'll develop Alzheimer's. Many people have one (or even two) copies of the gene and never get the disease. Conversely, some people don't have any copies of the ApoE4 gene and still develop Alzheimer's. We're looking at relative risks, not guarantees. Give it some thought and decide whether you want to peer into this crystal ball.

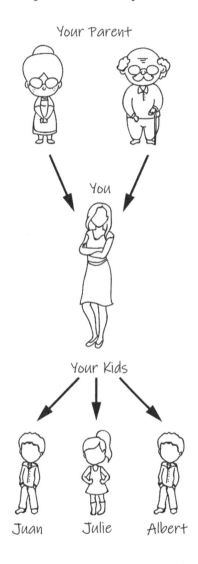

Zinc - Zinc deficiency is a common problem worldwide. People with low zinc levels are at greater risk for chronic inflammation and insulin dysfunction. Low zinc levels may accelerate aging and increase your risk for Alzheimer's disease. There is some evidence that zinc may reduce your risk of the common cold. Zinc is particularly important for sports nutrition. The mineral plays a role in athletic performance, recovery, and testosterone production. Unfortunately, athletes' zinc levels often run too low. Your goal red blood cell zinc level is 12-14 mg/dL. [Note: zinc appears to be protective from respiratory viruses similar to COVID-19. Taking high doses of zinc (75 mg/day) for the first five days of symptoms might reduce the duration and severity of the common cold and the Coronavirus.]

Tissue transglutaminase (TTG) and deamidated gliadin peptide (DGP) - Celiac disease is an autoimmune disorder caused by your body's abnormally strong reaction to gluten. The immune system of folks with celiac disease gets revved up when it detects gluten and goes on a rampage, causing inflammation and damaging tissues throughout the body. The intestines and brain are often the hardest hit. Chronic inflammation contributes to aging. Common symptoms of celiac disease are diarrhea, abdominal pain, mood disturbances, depression, anemia, and osteoporosis. Some people with celiac disease have no outward symptoms but suffer internal damage. The TTG and DGP labs are easy blood tests to screen for celiac disease.

ESR and CRP - One of the recurring themes of this book and aging research in general is that chronic inflammation is bad news. Your normal cells are innocent victims in the crossfire of your inflamed immune system run amok. As discussed elsewhere in this chapter, people with periodontal disease (swelling and inflammation of the gums) are at increased risk for heart disease. The body is interconnected, and problems in one area can cause trouble everywhere. The ESR and CRP tests are markers for systemic inflammation. They may indicate a chronic problem (like an autoimmune disorder) or they may signify something acute and minor, like a recent cold or infection. While the tests aren't perfect, it is worth monitoring them and following their levels over time. Your goal is to have them be as low as possible.

Measure your omega 3 levels

I hope by now that I've convinced you that omega-3 fatty acids are important for your health and wellness. High levels of omega-3 fatty acids are good for your heart, brain, eyes, and overall inflammation. They appear to reduce the risk of depression, rheumatoid arthritis, cancer, and Alzheimer's disease.

The trouble is, just like resveratrol, you need to get and keep the omega-3s in your body for them to do their thing. It's great to eat fish, flax seeds, and chia, but if you aren't absorbing and retaining enough omega-3s, you haven't done your job.

So, how do you know if you have enough omega-3s? It turns out that there's a simple test. Companies like OmegaQuant will measure the omega-3 fatty acid profile of your red blood cells. You don't even need to go to the lab. They'll send you a kit and you draw the blood yourself with a tiny finger prick. Some of their packages will even test your omega-6 and trans-fat levels.

Once you know your omega-3 level, you can make personalized dietary changes. See the theme here? If your omega-3 level is low, it may be that your twice-weekly tuna burgers aren't enough. You might need to add some more salmon, sardines, omega-3 supplements, seaweed, walnuts, and algae.

On the other hand, if your omega-3 levels are high, you can pat yourself on the back for a job well done. You're likely to have a longer and healthier life.

This test may also have value for pregnant women or nursing mothers. If your omega-3 levels are higher, your baby will benefit from improved levels of this health-promoting fat.

Speak with your obstetrician about omega-3s and pregnancy, as you want to give your baby an ample supply of omega-3s but you don't want to expose them to too much mercury (which can be found in some fish).

PART III

Lifestyle, technology, and wellness

Dental Health

When you think about important organs in your body, you probably think of your heart and brain. If you're a little more adventurous, perhaps you think of your kidneys and liver. But, do you ever consider your gums?

You should.

It turns out that your gums are a key to your overall health. When your mouth is sick, it will drag your whole body down with it. The connection between your gums and body is more dramatic and dangerous than you think. Modern research links periodontal disease (gum disease) to:

- Alzheimer's disease
- Complications during pregnancy
- Osteoporosis
- Cancer
- Heart disease
- Stroke

As you can see, all the above conditions are serious hallmarks of aging. Since the goal of this book is to keep you young and virile, we need to ward off these age-related conditions.

Here's the deal. Your teeth are covered with a nasty biofilm called plaque. Plaque is a sticky slime loaded with tons of hungry bacteria. They love nothing more than to feast on your sugary meals of soda and candy bars. With time, plaque can harden into tartar at the gumline. Tartar, along with all the associated bacteria, releases toxins and irritates your gums and causes gingivitis. Gingivitis, or gum inflammation, is characterized by redness and mild swelling. Gingivitis is a sign that your gums are starting to suffer from the nasty germs in your mouth.

If left untreated, gingivitis will turn into the more severe periodontitis, with bleeding gums (during brushing or at the dentist), bright red or purplish color changes, pain, and bad breath. With time, your gums will recede or pull away from your teeth and your teeth will loosen as you lose the supportive bone under your gums.

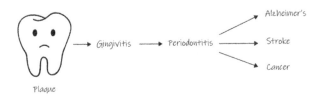

Gum disease, inflammation, and the diseases of aging

What causes gum disease? Here's a partial list of causes adapted from the Mayo Clinic:

- Poor self-care of your teeth including inadequate brushing, flossing, and dental visits
- Smoking and chewing tobacco

- Certain medications, including those that dry your mouth (like some antidepressants)
- Hormonal changes
- Age
- Obesity
- Poor nutrition
- Stress
- Weakened immune system from chemotherapy, cancer, and HIV
- Autoimmune diseases like rheumatoid arthritis and Crohn's disease
- Chronic high blood sugar, as in poorly-controlled diabetes

You're probably thinking, why would gum problems cause so much trouble for the rest of my body? It's just the mouth, right?

Good question. One of the key takeaways from this book is that your whole body is interconnected. Western medicine makes the mistake of over-compartmentalizing things. Your kidneys, brain, lungs, and, yes, gums, don't just exist in a vacuum. They all work together to make the whole you. When part of your body suffers, your whole body suffers.

In the case of your teeth and gums, there are a couple of theories as to why gum disease wreaks havoc on the rest of your body.

Bacteria leak through your gums and travel throughout your body. The bacteria *P. gingivalis* is one of the main pathogens in gum disease. Scientists discovered that this germ can actually sneak past the gums and travel to the brain. This nasty germ seems to play a role in Alzheimer's disease. It appears to travel to the placenta in pregnant women, endangering the fetus.

Our old friend, inflammation, is one of the key drivers of aging. Chronic bacterial infections in your gums rev up your immune system. Your overactive oral immune system releases nasty cytokines, or chemical messengers that dial-up inflammation throughout your body. Indeed, *P. gingivalis* has been shown to increase the body's level of inflammatory substances like TNF-α and IL-6. Once your body's immune system is turned on, it starts going crazy by releasing toxic substances and harming normal tissues. It is this excessive immune response, or systemic inflammation, which is believed to contribute to cancer, heart disease, and other illnesses of aging.

What can you do? Simple, take good care of your teeth. Here are some basic rules to keep your mouth, and the rest of your body, healthy.

Brush and floss every day. Make sure you brush at least twice a day for at least two minutes each time. Brush by the gumline. Use a soft-bristled toothbrush and replace it regularly, before the bristles are all bent and nasty.

Make regular trips to your dentist.

Use mouthwash. I prefer the kinds without alcohol because the alcohol seems to dry out my mouth. Ask your dentist which brands they recommend.

Avoid sugary meals. Sugar feeds the bad germs on your teeth and increases inflammation throughout your body. If you must eat sugar, do your best to brush your teeth right after.

Avoid medicines that dry out your mouth.

Manage your blood sugar. Do your best to keep it in the low-normal range.

Don't smoke or use chewing tobacco.

Reduce your stress levels. Meditate and practice mindfulness, gratitude, and tai chi.

Eat healthy foods. Proper nutrition is good for gums and will increase your levels of healthy bacteria.

Your beautiful teeth won't just land you your next modeling gig, they'll keep you out of the nursing home.

Mood and ketamine

Mental pain is less dramatic than physical pain, but it is more common and also more hard to bear. The frequent attempt to conceal mental pain increases the burden: it is easier to say "My tooth is aching" than to say "My heart is broken.

~C.S. Lewis

Your mental wellbeing cannot play second-fiddle to your physical health. When you're struggling with depression, self-doubt, or anxiety, nothing else seems very important.

That's why I urge you to take your mental health seriously. Don't ignore depression and don't depend on the assessments of your friends and coworkers. See a mental health professional and try the wellness suggestions in this book.

For those who still suffer from depression despite trying antidepressants, there is hope. Ketamine is a powerful and effective antidepressant that can work in as little as one treatment.

Ketamine is often successful even when other medications fail. Many people with nowhere else to turn found relief and rejuvenation from ketamine therapy. When administered by an anesthesiologist or psychiatrist trained in its use, ketamine can be a lifesaver.

As time goes on, I suspect that more and more people will turn to ketamine to improve their mood and drive. Unlike antidepressants, it doesn't require daily use. You escape the side effects of the other antidepressants including sexual dysfunction and weight gain. And for some people, a few treatments (and, perhaps, an occasional booster) might be all you need for a lifetime of mental health.

Beyond ketamine, many of the other tips in this chapter will improve mood, drive, energy, and focus. I've personally found that I'm more energetic and productive when I fast. Heavy meals sap your energy, and intermittent fasting is a simple solution. Skip out on the blood sugar roller coaster, it's no good for your mood or spirit.

Omega 3s, coffee, adequate sleep, metformin, exercise, testosterone replacement, and vitamin D, zinc, and light therapy are all proven mood and energy boosters.

If you're reluctant to take pills for your depression, why don't you start out by examining elements of your health that you can easily control? Get more quality sleep. Get checked for sleep apnea. Enjoy more salmon and wholesome olive oil. Go to the gym, run, swim, or play tennis 3-4 times a week. Make these simple changes and you may find that you feel better without the need for drugs.

Even if you are one of the lucky few who benefit from typical antidepressant drugs, I still urge you to try the other wellness techniques listed in this chapter. You'll increase your energy and sharpen your focus. You might even find (in consultation with your mental health professional) that you no longer need to take antidepressants.

Your brain, body, health, diet, sleep, mood, and vigor are all interconnected. Your sense of wellbeing and your body aren't like separate planets each orbiting their own sun. Rather, your physical and mental health are intimately related.

I mention depression in this chapter because scientists believe that depression is aging. Remarkably, your cells respond to your mood. Major depression is associated with short telomeres.

It's a tragic mistake that Western medicine compartmentalizes our body parts rather than considering the whole you. We aren't just a big sack carrying a heart, brain, liver, etc. We are a unified being and each part of us connects and impacts everything else. The tips here will benefit your whole self, your body, and your mind.

Technology

Tech is one of my favorite weapons in the war on aging. I routinely employ a variety of the most cutting-edge technological gizmos to create a customized wellness plan for my patients.

I'd like to share a few of the technological tools I use with you here. However, since technology is constantly changing, I'll only mention the categories of devices rather than specific brands. Any particular device I mention today may be out of date by the time you read this book. To keep up with my favorite technology products, be sure to visit my website. Dr. Peter Attia also has great content on technology.

These are the classes of technology I recommend, most of which I use to optimize my wellness patients:

Continuous glucose monitor (CGM) - You already know about this one. When combined with a dietary log, the CGM is the most powerful tool available to create a customized meal plan tailored for your body.

At-home sleep apnea test - Obstructive sleep apnea is a killer. It ages you, drains your energy, and increases your risk of heart disease and Alzheimer's. If you have untreated sleep apnea, you'll perform worse in school, at work, and on the field. And with today's technology, it's so easy to find out whether you have OSA. There are some fantastic home sleep tests that will diagnose OSA with a high degree of reliability. These gizmos will measure your sleep quality, oxygen levels, respiratory distress, time sleeping, and movement. A one-night test in the comfort of your own bedroom might add years to your life. You may also want to consider other sleep optimizing devices like rings and watches.

Neurofeedback devices - There are many new devices, many of which were unveiled at CES, that measure your brainwaves or EEG to help you master your mind. There are cutting-edge tools that will improve your sleep quality and efficiency. There are new non-pharmacologic treatments for anxiety and depression. Elite athletes will benefit from monitors that measure and improve focus at the gym. There are similar tools that can improve your concentration while working or studying. These devices are your secret weapon for business success. You can even peer into your brain to improve the quality of your meditation.

"Continuous" at-home blood pressure monitors - I'm excited about this technology. Here's the issue. Doctors will diagnose you with high blood pressure (HTN) and start you on powerful, life-long medications based on a couple of abnormal blood pressure (BP) readings in their office. I don't blame them for treating HTN, after all, it is linked to heart disease and stroke. The trouble is that I'm not sure we're diagnosing it correctly. For example, your readings in the doctor's office might be high because you're anxious. This phenomenon is often called "white coat hypertension." They could also be high because you were rushing and running late to the appointment, you had to climb stairs to get to the office, or the cuff was placed or sized incorrectly. Do we really want to commit you to a lifetime of medications (and side effects) based on a few sloppy measurements?

The other problem with the current system is that we don't honestly know whether the blood pressure medication is working properly. Once you start the medicine, your only follow-up will be a couple of readings in the office. We're back in the same boat. Once again, we're depending on a few shoddy and unreliable measurements without knowing whether your treatment is actually working. Did we lower your BP enough? Did we overshoot and lower it too much?

Now, welcome to the wonderful world of home blood pressure monitoring. While the technology is still being worked out, it is now possible to take dozens or hundreds of BP readings in your home. We'll see your BP while you're eating dinner, watching TV, and reading the news. We'll know for sure if you have HTN. And we'll know whether you're responding appropriately to your medication. It will be easy to make the right changes to optimize your health and extend your life.

Ketone monitors - For those of you practicing prolonged fasting or ketogenic diets, I recommend you purchase a ketone monitor or test strips. You want to chart your progress, make sure you're achieving ketosis, and watch that you're not going overboard.

At-home skin cancer detection - Skin cancer is one of the most common types of cancer, with an estimated one in five people suffering from the disease. The good news is that most skin cancers are easily treated if you catch them early. That's the trick. Unfortunately, many of us ignore potentially problematic lesions and wait too long to get checked. We don't want to spend hours going to the doctor's office only to be told that we have a mole or age spot. Now, there is a solution. There are skin cancer apps for your phone that use artificial intelligence to evaluate all your suspicious moles. You just take a picture of anything concerning, and powerful computers will determine whether you need to go to the doctor's office for a complete examination. Early skin cancer detection is key, and these new apps may just save your life.

Activity trackers - Are you getting your steps? While the truth is that a few steps here and there don't match up with moderate to high-intensity exercise, fitness trackers play a role. They motivate you to walk more and create a culture around exercise. Plus, it's fun to see how many steps you've taken. They can be particularly useful for seniors, people with disabilities, and corporations. Seniors and those with injuries that limit their ability to exercise reap enormous benefits from walking and taking the stairs compared with being sedentary. It turns out that some exercise is far better than none. Corporations are using fitness trackers to incentivize their employees to exercise. The data is clear on this one, a fit workforce uses fewer sick days, is more productive, and saves money on health insurance costs. I recommend all my corporate clients, particularly those who provide health insurance, to encourage the use of fitness/activity trackers.

TENS - Transcutaneous electrical nerve stimulation, or TENS for short, treats pain without medication. It uses low-voltage electric currents to block the pain signal between the irritated part of the body to the brain. It appears to dial-down your pain response and restores your body's natural ability to fight pain. TENS can be used to treat pain in the neck, back, bones, and joints. Pregnant women in labor and people with cancer often enjoy relief from TENS units. As an anesthesiologist, I'm particularly excited about how effective TENS can be for postoperative pain. TENS is also great for athletes with sports-related injuries.

For some people with chronic pain, a brief TENS treatment yields prolonged pain relief. Think about that. A few zaps for electricity and you're off pain pills and feeling great. Others may need to use TENS for a while to treat their pain. It appears to be safe and free of side effects. A successful TENS treatment can wean someone off pain medication, improve mood, and eliminate pain-related depression. When we treat pain, folks who couldn't exercise can now go back out there and work on their fitness. TENS is anti-aging because it increases exercise, reduces inflammation, and likely lengthens telomeres by uplifting mood and reducing stress.

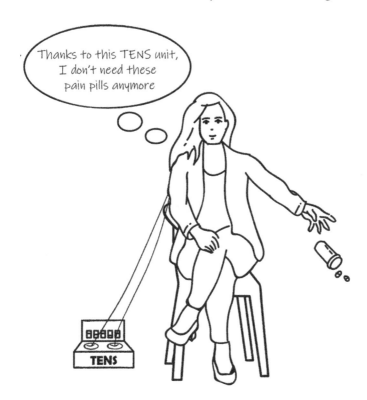

TENS units can treat pain without drugs

Thanks to this TENS unit, I don't need these pain pills anymore

Seek sun exposure (without going overboard) and avoid radiation

The sun is a double-edged sword. A study of 30,000 women in Europe found that those with limited sun exposure experienced a two-fold greater risk of early death. You read that right. Sun exposure reduces all-cause mortality. It is a mistake to spend all day indoors.

[Author's note: I included this study in the reference section for your review. Don't worry, it's pretty easy to read. Although the study looked at an impressive 30,000 people prospectively for a total of over 500,000 person-years, it does have some serious limitations which cause me to question its accuracy. For one, it isn't randomized. That means that the study participants sorted themselves out into the high-sun and low-sun groups. It could be that the low-sun people were sicker, more obese, or less active independent of their sun exposure. It is also based on surveys, and people are notoriously inaccurate with questionnaires. Think about the last time you filled out a form some stranger gave you about your lifestyle. In summary, more research is needed on this critical topic.]

There are some good reasons to believe that sun exposure will improve your health. Your skin needs the sun to create the active form of vitamin D, a critical nutrient that most of us lack. It's a good bet that your vitamin D levels are low. Sun exposure, particularly in the morning, helps maintain a proper circadian rhythm. People who stay indoors all day are less likely to exercise. And, sun (along with outdoor green-spaces) improves mood and battles depression.

You officially have my blessing to enjoy some rays.

The trouble with the sun is that most studies show excessive exposure increases your risk for skin cancer, cataracts, wrinkles, and DNA damage which can cause premature aging. Chronic excessive sun exposure dramatically increases your risk for basal and squamous cell skin cancer. Sunburns, particularly during childhood, increase your risk for a potentially deadly melanoma.

The sun contains ultraviolet radiation, which, as we'll see in a moment, is no good for your DNA. I recommend that you check the UV index before you go outdoors for any prolonged period. You can easily find it online or on your phone's weather app. A low UV index (under 3) means that you can enjoy the outdoors with less concern for skin cancer. If the UV index is high, I recommend limiting your time outside. If you must be out during the risky midafternoon period, be sure to wear protective clothes, sunglasses, and mineral-based sunscreen. You should also note that clouds aren't so great at blocking harmful UV rays—so you shouldn't be complacent just because it's an overcast day.

While the sun may have its benefits, the story with radiation is all bad. Radiation exposure increases your risk of cancer and early death, particularly for children. The location and type of cancer depend on the type of radiation. And the amount of increased risk depends on the quantity of radiation (measured in mSv) and your age at the time of exposure.

Radiation will make you old.

Here's the deal. Radiation comes flying through your cells, crashing into your DNA. This direct frontal assault on your genes breaks the DNA apart and introduces errors. Radiation indirectly attacks your DNA by creating dangerous and highly active free radicals right next to your chromosomes. These free radicals go around tearing apart your DNA, resulting in mutations, cell death, and senescence.

As we shared earlier, accumulating too many senescent cells will age you. They clog up the works, impair tissue and immune performance, and create inflammation. DNA damage can create mutant cells that evolve into cancer. Finally, the DNA damage will short circuit your sirtuin longevity pathways, weakening your defenses against the ravages of time.

By causing your body to accumulate senescent cells, create mutant and potentially cancerous cells, and by impairing your youth-promoting sirtuins, radiation is all bad news. Our goal is to minimize your exposure.

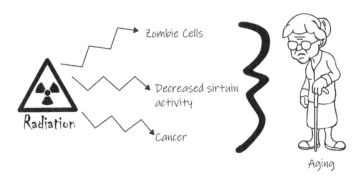

The most common sources of radiation are medical sources and radon gas. X-rays, CT scans, and some nuclear medicine studies are the main culprits.

Here is a table of relative radiation exposure from various sources adapted from data shared by the University of Wisconsin. The goal of this table is to compare various sources of radiation to how much radiation you'd get from one x-ray. For the purpose of this table, the radiation exposure from an x-ray is considered "1 unit" and everything else is a multiple of that 1.

Table 2. Quantity of radiation by source compared with a standard x-ray

Source	Approximate relative radiation exposure
x-ray	1
Mammogram	5
CT Scan	20-200
Nuclear cardiac stress test	400
Airport body scanner (millimeter-wave scanner)	0.001
10-hour plane flight	1
Annual radiation exposure living at high altitudes (ie. Denver)	5

While I worry about the radiation exposure from medical imaging, sometimes you just need those exams. I am not advocating that you never get an x-ray, CT scan, etc. However, you should avoid unnecessary studies. Go ahead and ask your doctor whether there is a safer alternative to your CT scans, such as an MRI or ultrasound. Let them know that you'd like to avoid radiation whenever possible.

[Author's note: There is some interesting new research about radiation exposure and hormesis. As you recall, the concept of hormesis is that a small amount of a stressor is actually good for you, while large doses are dangerous. Radiation hormesis postulates that a bit of radiation exposure (like living in high-altitude cities like Denver), might actually be beneficial. Perhaps this minor stressor ramps up your body's cellular repair systems. There is no dispute, however, that large amounts of radiation are toxic. Stay tuned to more research on this fascinating topic.]

Radon is an odorless and colorless gas that may be responsible for 21,000 lung cancer deaths per year according to the EPA. The risk of lung cancer from radon is increased in smokers, but 3,000 people die from radon-induced lung cancer who never smoked.

Radon is found in buildings and homes—possibly yours. It seeps in from the ground and the only way to know whether your home has radon is to get it tested. Do-it-yourself radon testing kits are easy and affordable. If your house has radon, there are some options you can do to reduce your exposure. There's no excuse, go out and get tested.

Red light

You go to the spa after work. But instead of a dip in the whirlpool or a trip to the massage table, you enter a special chamber. The attendant flips a switch and you're bathed in the warm glow of a deep, red light. You emerge after 12 minutes, rejuvenated.

You just enjoyed one of the hottest trends in wellness medicine (pun intended), red light therapy.

Red and infrared light appears to have a variety of health benefits. Although the research on red light therapy (RLT) isn't as comprehensive as it is for some other practices mentioned here, RLT is worth your time and may improve your life. I recommend it to most of my clients who are professional athletes and anyone looking to remain young. Here are some of the benefits:

Treats injuries - It appears to speed up wound healing, support bone recovery, and decrease pain.

Improves sleep and athletic performance - Studies suggest soccer and basketball players benefit from targeted RLT to improve sleep quality and enhance their athletic performance. This is particularly true for those who travel or have training schedules at off-hours. It also seems to enhance muscle recovery for football players.

Anti-aging - It appears to decrease inflammation, increase heat shock proteins, and triggers your body to remove unwanted cells.

You'll look better - RLT increases collagen production in your skin, thereby reducing the appearance of fine lines and wrinkles. RLT may decrease acne, help regrow hair, and improve the appearance of burns and surgical scars.

If you're interested in trying RLT, I recommend you go to a gym, medical spa, wellness center, or dermatologist who offers the service. You can purchase a package of several treatments and see how you like it. If you fall in love with the device, you can even buy a modified version for home.

Meditation, mindfulness, and gratitude

Brilliant author and forefather of lifestyle design, Tim Ferriss, is famous for the company he keeps. In his book *Tools of Titans,* Ferriss interviews some of the world's top performers. The men and women in the book are elite athletes, successful politicians, business executives, and celebrities. He asks each of them to share the secrets of their success. What do most of them mention? Meditation and mindfulness.

If meditation can boost Arnold Schwarzenegger's game, it will boost yours.

It turns out that Schwarzenegger and Ferriss were on to something. Each day, more and more research proves the deep and lasting value of meditation and mindfulness.

Before we go into the benefits, I'd like to briefly describe these practices.

Meditation - There are many types of meditation, and I cannot do justice to this rich and valuable topic in a few lines here. Meditation typically involves relaxation, focus, body awareness, and love. I strongly recommend that you read some books dedicated to meditation or speak with a meditation practitioner. If you're looking for a high-tech solution, Calm and Headspace are popular smartphone apps that will walk you through the basics of meditation.

Mindfulness - Mindfulness is the opposite of multitasking. The goal here is to be present in the moment and focus on what you're doing. Don't think about tomorrow's work presentation while you're in the yard playing catch with your daughter.

Gratitude - The practice of gratitude is the intentional act of being thankful when good things happen or when someone does something nice for you. The goal is to help you appreciate the good in others and to prevent you from taking things for granted. Each night before bed, my kids and I share our favorite moments of the day. They can be large (I'm glad we made it home safely from our trip) or small (I'm thankful that my friend shared her pencil with me at school when I lost mine). Many people keep a gratitude journal and list five or ten things that happened over the day that they appreciate. Gratitude forces us to focus on the good rather than fixate on the bad. As I always tell my kids, "What do you think will make you a happier person, focusing on the game you lost last night or on tomorrow's big visit with Grandma?"

Breathwork - There are certain breathing exercises that are proven to reduce stress, increase focus, improve mood, decrease blood pressure, and enhance meditation. They're often easy to do and they don't take much time - you can easily fit them in your schedule. Going back to my kids, when they spill a drink on the chair for the 100th time, I make a habit of stopping and taking a slow, deep breath before I lose my cool. I find that that one breath calms me down and prevents me from overreacting. Breathing techniques like Wim Hof, Lion's Breath, and deep breathing calm the spirit and reduce stress. There are some great apps to encourage your breathwork practice.

Certain exercises - Yoga, tai chi, and qigong all have tons of health benefits. They're accessible to folks of any age and physical condition. I suggest you attend a class, meet with an experienced practitioner, or watch some online videos to experience these life-promoting exercises.

I advise you to experiment with all of these practices and see which ones work best for you. I'll probably find that you enjoy a variety of meditative practices, and you'll want to combine them to achieve maximum benefit. Speaking of benefits, here are some of the proven reasons why you need to start your meditation practice today:

Telomeres - You read that right. Meditation and mindfulness will actually lengthen your telomeres (see below). Meditation also decreases inflammation and combats aging. Practice tai chi and your cells will thank you. You may have to stock up on some more birthday candles.

Reduced stress - Stress is one of the leading killers. It causes headaches, muscle tension, fatigue, decreased sex drive, sleep disorders, irregular eating, and anger. Stress weakens your immune system, increases your blood sugar (bad), and likely increases your risk for heart disease and stroke. Nip stress in the bud with mindfulness.

Meditation improves work performance and job satisfaction - This is why many of the most successful people regularly meditate. If you're an executive, I recommend that you encourage your employees to meditate and practice mindfulness. You'll boost their productivity and collaboration. Who doesn't want happy employees?

Improved gut bacteria (microbiome) - Everyone is talking about the importance of a healthy microbiome, and for good reason. When you have a rich variety of beneficial organisms living in your gut, you'll have fewer colds, more energy, and a lower risk for autoimmune diseases. A healthy gut microbiome may also reduce your risk of depression. And here's the kicker. It seems that stress doesn't just hurt you, it adversely impacts the microorganisms living in your intestines. When you're stressed, you may be killing off the beneficial bacteria that you need to keep healthy. Fortunately, stress reduction via meditative practices may improve your intestinal microbiome and boost your overall health.

Connection to others is an essential component of mindfulness, life satisfaction, and telomere health. While it's important to focus inward for self-improvement and reflection, make sure you also send love outward to aid friends, neighbors, family, and the less fortunate in your community.

Cryotherapy

While this won't appeal to everyone, cryotherapy might be one of the easiest, safest, and fashionable ways to boost your health.

Here's the idea. You step into a freezing chamber often wearing nothing more than your underpants. After three or four minutes you emerge, mentally refreshed and physically recharged. Athletes (and Kevin Hart) are known to take ice baths. Alternatively, you can do simplified (and cheaper) versions of cryotherapy by taking walks through the snow in a t-shirt, eating your lunch outside on a cold day, and allowing your bedroom to cool down when you sleep.

It's thought that cryotherapy works by increasing your body's production of brown fat. Unlike the unsavory white fat that we're all trying to lose, brown fat is chocked full of mitochondria, your cell's energy factories. These busy little cells and their over-achieving mitochondria will burn calories for you all day and, hopefully, help you lose weight.

Some researchers believe that cryotherapy reduces inflammation. You're reading this book because you want to fight aging. If you can reduce your chronic inflammation and achieve a healthy weight, you've won most of the battle. Beyond weight loss, there are anecdotal reports that cryotherapy reduces muscle and migraine pain, fights depression, and alleviates eczema.

I should note that while a lot of athletes practice cryotherapy, it should not be considered a tool for increasing muscle mass. In fact, active recovery (like swimming, light resistance training, hiking, and yoga) is superior to cryotherapy for muscle development. Rather, you should use cryo for weight loss, decreasing inflammation, reducing muscle pain, and natural rejuvenation.

If you want to try cryotherapy, maximize your benefits by following it with productive work. Take advantage of the invigoration and crank out some good stuff in the office. After cryo, go tackle that screenplay or report you've been putting off. It might be better (gasp) than a cup of coffee.

Telomeres

Telomeres are drawing a lot of attention in the press and medical journals thanks to groundbreaking work by Dr. Elizabeth Blackburn and colleagues. For those interested in this topic, I encourage you to read her book, *The Telomere Effect.* Here's a brief overview of what telomeres are and why they're relevant for aging.

Generic material called DNA resides in nearly all of our cells. The genes in DNA call the shots. They code for all the different proteins manufactured by your body and determine your eye color, blood type, and even how you metabolize toxins. Human DNA is partitioned into 46 different structures called chromosomes. Think of chromosomes as tightly packed spools of DNA ready to spring into action as new proteins are required.

At the tips of each chromosome are segments of DNA called telomeres. The telomere's job is to protect the structure of the chromosome. It does not code for protein. Rather, the telomere is there to make sure the rest of the chromosome remains structurally intact during cellular replication.

As we discussed, you can think of the telomere as the little plastic bit on the end of a shoelace. That small plastic piece prevents the shoelace from unraveling and falling apart. The telomere does the same for your chromosome.

Cells in your body are constantly turning over. Over the natural course of life, cells die and need to be replaced. New cells are manufactured when you grow, suffer an injury, or when conditions change. Our cells and bodies are dynamic.

The process we use to produce new cells is called mitosis. Mitosis is the scientific name for when one parent cell splits into two identical daughter cells. To ensure that each of the daughter cells has her own complete set of DNA, the parent cell makes a copy of its DNA—one copy for each daughter cell.

Here's where the telomeres come in. Each time a cell divides through mitosis, it's possible that the telomere can lose a little bit of length. It is as though that small plastic cap at the end of your shoelaces shrinks a bit every time your chromosome is copied. Eventually, the telomeres grow so short that a cell can no longer copy itself correctly. The cell is old.

Many scientists view the length of telomeres as a sign of cellular aging. The shorter the telomeres, the older the cell. Telomere shortening is one of the three causes of aging, along with epigenetic changes and the accumulation of zombie (senescent) cells.

If you're in the camp that believes that telomere length is a proxy for cellular aging, then one of the goals of anti-aging medicine should be to protect and preserve telomeres. It turns out that certain lifestyle choices, chemical exposures, and even psychological states can damage your telomeres.

In other words, not everyone's telomeres will shrink at the same rate. Environmental and lifestyle factors will cause your telomeres to shrink at a different pace than mine. Therefore, your cells and my cells will age at different speeds. Our job here is to pump the breaks on our cellular aging.

Here is a list of some known causes of telomere shortening and cellular aging:

Chronic, toxic stress. For example, an abusive relationship, food and housing insecurity, and fear of physical violence

• Physical and emotional trauma

• Depression, particularly severe depression. This is another reason to treat depression - since depression can cause you to age

• Caregiving for an ill dependent

• Highly stressful work environments

• Loneliness and isolation

• Smoking. Another reason to quit.

• Eating processed meats (hotdogs, sandwich meats, ham)

• Sugar

• Chemical exposures including air pollution (i.e. living near a major road), certain pesticides, lead, benzene, arsenic, and exposures from chemicals and gasses in a car mechanic's workshop

• Sleep deprivation. Here is yet another example of the importance of sleep

And here are some things you can do to preserve your telomeres and potentially fight cellular aging:

• Regular exercise. Shoot for aerobic exercise at least 45 minutes three times a week

• Eat real foods like veggies, fruit, and whole grains. In particular, eat as many veggies as possible. Shoot for a variety of colors.

• Meditation, mindfulness, and gratitude

• Exposure to green spaces like parks and forests

• A strong social network of family, neighbors, and friends

• Restorative practices like qigong and Tai Chi

• Meet your neighbors, participate in social activities, and reconnect with your family

For those who are interested, there are commercially available tests for telomere length. They can help you get a sense of your DNA health and cellular age. However, I don't recommend them at this point. The tests are not regulated and have questionable accuracy. Moreover, their results are not easy to interpret and have unclear predictive value. Rather than take a telomere test, I suggest you do anything you can to reduce your exposure to the telomere toxins on the first list and enhance your exposure to healthful telomere promoters on list two.

Sleep and OSA

I won't bore you to sleep (see what I did there) by discussing sleep too much here since we cover sleep in another chapter. But since this chapter is about increasing your health span and improving your longevity, I want to focus on how sleep keeps you young.

When you deprive yourself of adequate sleep, you're taking a wrecking ball to your cells. You can age yourself with just one night of bad sleep. If you're like me and want to remain young and vigorous, sleep is some serious stuff. Here are some of the scientifically-proven ways that inadequate sleep will make you old.

- Sleep deprivation shortens your telomeres. As you recall, short telomeres are a marker for cellular aging. Multiple studies confirm the link between sleep and telomere length. Here are some of the findings:
  - o Shorter telomeres in patients with obstructive sleep apnea (OSA)
  - o Fetuses had shorter telomeres when mom had an OSA variant called sleep-disordered breathing
  - o Women with poor sleep quality had shorter telomeres.
  - o Men with short sleep duration suffered shorter telomeres.
  - o Older adults with adequate sleep enjoyed longer telomeres than their sleep-deprived peers.

- As little as one night of partial sleep deprivation appears to increase cellular senescence (increased expression of NFKB2 and DNA damage response signals). As you recall, large numbers of senescent cells are both a marker for and a cause of aging. You want to keep these naughty zombie cells to a minimum.

- Improper sleep, including OSA, increases inflammation, decreases immune function, causes epigenetic changes (which are one of the key drivers of aging), and harms stem cells.

- Sleep deprivation increases the risk of diseases associated with the elderly including Alzheimer's, heart disease, stroke, and cancer.

The older you are, the harder it is to get a good night's sleep. Seniors tend to have altered sleep-wake cycles, more nighttime arousals (bathroom trips), and decreased REM and deep NREM sleep. It can be tougher to fall asleep and even harder to stay asleep. This natural sleep disturbance with age can lead to a vicious cycle. You age, then you sleep worse, then your poor sleep makes you age faster. Your job is to break this dangerous cycle.

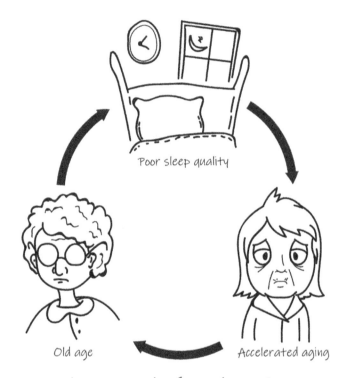

Poor sleep quality

Old age

Accelerated aging

The vicious cycle of poor sleep and aging

Follow the recommendations in the sleep chapter to improve the quantity and quality of your shuteye.

One final note about OSA. If you have it, you must get treated. Even if you are in bed for a solid eight hours, if you're gasping for air all night, you won't achieve the deep, restorative sleep your body requires. Your telomeres will shrink and your cells will suffer. You'll age prematurely, increase your risk of disability, and die sooner. If you snore, get tested and treated.

Regular exercise

You didn't think I was going to let you off the hook with exercise, did you? In addition to a healthy diet and proper sleep, regular exercise is one of the best things you can do for your health. No amount of fish oil or oregano will make up for sitting on the couch all day watching reality TV. You need to get out there and work those muscles.

You want to stay young, energic, and vigorous? Are you looking to forestall the ravages and illnesses of the elderly? Your answer is simple. Exercise.

Exercise is anti-aging.

As discussed earlier, your body has all sorts of longevity and age-fighting pathways. Regular exercise engages your longevity genes and proteins. Your trips to the gym, swimming pool, tennis courts, and mountain trails train your age-regulating systems like AMPK and the sirtuins to work in your favor. Exercise also pumps up your NAD levels, a fountain of youth for your cells.

Regular aerobic exercise increases telomere length. As we discussed earlier, telomere length is a marker for cellular aging and DNA health. When you work up a sweat, you're strengthening your genes. Those brisk walks aren't just pumping up your glutes, they're changing your body chemistry to keep you young.

Here are some additional benefits of regular exercise:

- You're less likely to die. An investigation of 120,000 people found that improved fitness resulted in substantially lower rates of death during the study period. The greater the fitness, the better the health.
- Reduced risk of depression
- Weight loss. Exercise burns calories, regulates your appetite, and increases your muscle mass.

Your extra muscle burns calories 24/7 - even while you sleep.

- Reduced risk of heart attack and stroke
- Stronger bones. Strength and impact exercise help prevent osteoporosis.
- Better sleep. Exercise (except right before bedtime) increases your sleep quantity and quality.
- Better sex. Regular exercise enhances sexual desire and performance.
- Lower risk of diabetes
- Lower risk of falls. Exercise increases your muscle strength and balance, reducing your risk of one of the most lethal accidents of the elderly.
- Improved workplace performance and productivity. Employers can boost their bottom line by encouraging their employees to exercise.

What exercise should you do and how often? I recommend that you shoot for at least 45 minutes of quality exercise at least three times a week. Aerobic interval training appears to be best for telomeres, but I strongly advise you to combine aerobic and strength training.

Aerobic exercise and weights (resistance or strength training) benefit your body in different and complementary ways. Jogging, swimming, and tennis are great for cardiovascular fitness, telomere length, and preventing depression. Resistance training is great for increasing muscle mass, preventing osteoporosis, and reducing your risk of falls. Both are great for promoting fat loss.

Two last points about exercise. First, there seems to be no upper limit for the benefit of exercise as long as you allow yourself adequate recovery periods. In other words, six days a week is better than three, provided you have some muscle recovery. Active recovery techniques like yoga and hikes are great on your days off.

Second, some exercise is better than nothing. Even one or two exercise days a week are better than sitting around on the couch (or spending all day at the office). Strolls around the park are good for you. Take the stairs, walk instead of drive, park far away, and work in your garden whenever you can. Your body, cells, and brain will thank you.

Now, let's move on to one of the most important determinants of health and aging—sleep.

Chapter 4

The Best Sleep of Your Life

Doctor Yohan Einstein threw his arms up in celebration. He finally did it. As the top scientist at Forever Young Pharmaceuticals, Dr. Einstein invented a pill to change the world.

When scholars took Dr. Einstein's pill after studying, their test scores skyrocketed. Armed with this new magical elixir, students actually remember their algebra and medieval history. They are more creative and successful in the classroom.

Bosses and managers using the pill are more popular and inspirational at work. The word is out: the new pill is the fast-track to the C Suite. Employees up and down the organization are more productive. They work better in teams and get more accomplished in less time. Workplace theft even declines.

Politicians are more charismatic, lawyers are more persuasive, and engineers crush their goals.

Athletes run faster, jump higher, and collaborate better with their teammates. Teams at the bottom of their divisions are suddenly in contention for the playoffs.

Drivers taking Dr. Einstein's pill are less likely to crash. Parents rest easier knowing that their teens are safe behind the wheel. In fact, road fatalities nearly disappear and auto insurance rates plummet.

Hospitals transform into ghost towns. Since the pill slashes the risk of cancer, viral respiratory infections, and Alzheimer's, people seldom need to go to the doctor.

To top it off, the pill even makes you look better.

Here's how it works: you simply take one tablet each evening. That's it. Oh, and there are no side-effects.

Okay, okay, the pill described above doesn't exist. But it doesn't have to. It turns out that you don't need a pill or Dr. Einstein to help you improve your memory, work performance, wakefulness, and health. You have everything you need right now at home: a pillow and a comfy blanket.

What is Dr. Einstein's pill? Consistent, high-quality, and sufficient sleep.

What is sleep?

Sleep is not the absence of wakefulness. It isn't just a period of downtime sandwiched between your daytime activities. Rather, sleep is a critical and highly-organized life function. Sleep is so important that it is preserved up and down the evolutionary ladder. Nearly every animal, including insects, birds, reptiles, and sea creatures sleep.

We all sleep because it is a necessary biological function. When you deprive nearly any animal of sleep it falls ill and dies. Dr. Matthew Walker has a wonderful explanation of the importance of sleep throughout the animal kingdom in his fantastic book, Why We Sleep (see bibliography).

Think about it for a moment. If sleep were no big deal, surely some animals would have evolved to live without it. If sleep were optional, there would be a huge competitive advantage to the fox, leopard, or wasp that could be active 24/7.

Imagine a "sleepless fox" named Billy. Sleep was completely unnecessary for him. He could hunt anytime, day or night. Since Billy never slept, he would always be aware of the surroundings and he'd be less likely to be killed by a hungry wolf. Nobody would sneak up on a sleeping Billy. And, our friend Billy would be a real Casanova, enjoying extra hours each day to woo the ladies. Billy would be the king of the foxes and his children would soon take over the fox community.

Yet, we have no sleepless foxes.

Billy, the sleepless fox

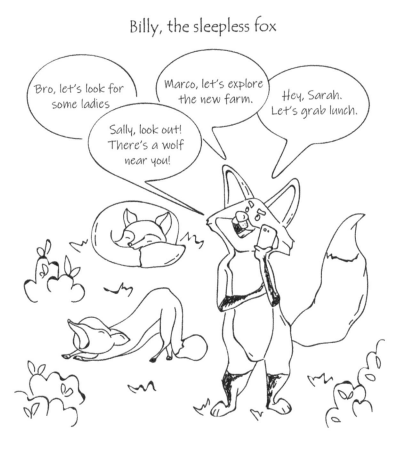

We have no sleepless foxes, birds, or beetles (bug sleep is called torpor) because sleep is essential for life.

Most mammalian sleep is divided into two distinct stages. The majority of the time is spent in a quiet non-rapid eye movement sleep (NREM) where the muscles are calm, the blood pressure and heart rate fall, and the body cools down. Your brainwaves during NREM sleep are regular, repeating, and highly-organized.

By contrast, rapid eye movement sleep (REM) is characterized by random and chaotic brainwaves. REM sleep is when you have your vivid and wild dreams. Did you ever imagine going to work without your pants? That was REM sleep. When you're in REM sleep, your eyes dart around but your muscles are flaccid and relaxed to prevent you from acting out all your crazy dreams.

The importance of sleep

If you're skimping on sleep, you're making a big mistake. Besides the obvious fact that you need sleep to live, here are some of the many health benefits of sleep:

Car crashes - You walk over to a friend's house and chit-chat late into the night. By the time you get home, it's already 3 a.m. Time flies. You jump in bed and snag four hours of sleep. The next morning, your alarm wrestles you awake. You dress and climb behind the wheel.

You never make it work.

When you sleep four hours or less, you're eleven times more likely to have a car accident. In fact, your risk of a car accident explodes with each extra hour of sleep deprivation below your required 7-8 hours.

Why does this happen? Microsleeps. You take these teeny-tiny naps behind the wheel when you're tired. For those brief moments, you are completely out of touch with the world—while driving a two-ton machine at 60 mph down the freeway. Bad news.

Alzheimer's disease - Alzheimer's is one of our most feared diseases. Scientists have long known that people with Alzheimer's disease usually have poor sleep. We are now starting to understand that poor sleep may be causing Alzheimer's disease. For example, we know that the sleep disturbance caused by shift work in midlife appears to increase the risk of dementia.

Why would poor sleep contribute to dementia? Recent research shows that your body actively removes the toxic, Alzheimer's-promoting chemicals tau and amyloid-beta during deep NREM sleep. When your slow-wave NREM sleep is disrupted (shift work, all-nighters, sleep apnea), you accumulate more of these dangerous chemicals in your brain. The buildup of these harmful substances may increase your risk of Alzheimer's. While the research on this is evolving (visit my website for the latest info) securing high-quality sleep might be your best bet for preventing this dreaded disease.

Emotional stability - You return home from a late family dinner and it is past bedtime. You unlock the door and your toddler, Sophie, bursts in and starts jumping all over the couches. She's giddy with excitement. Smiling, laughing, making froggy faces. Then, you tell her that it's late and you need to brush her teeth for bed. In a flash, her smile turns to tears. Sophie screams, yells, and collapses on the ground. It will be a tough night.

You've probably noticed the same thing about yourself. After a night of sleep deprivation, you're irritable. Your patience grows thin. Little things annoy you. Your mood darkens. Coworkers steer clear of you and your short fuse.

There's a scientific explanation for little Sophie's tantrums and your mood swings. Sleep deprivation causes the emotional control centers in your brain (the amygdala) to go haywire. You go start running around and acting out while your more rational cortical brain functions are asleep at the switch.

Attention and focus - Are you spacing out in class? Is it difficult for you to stay awake during your CFO's PowerPoint presentation on the year-end financials? It may be sleep deprivation. Research proves that you're less able to pay attention when you're sleep-deprived. This loss of focus happens even when you don't feel sleepy.

Obesity - We all know that marijuana gives you the munchies. It turns out that sleep-deprivation does too. When you don't get enough sleep, your body's production of the appetite-controlling hormones leptin and ghrelin is disturbed. As a result, your hunger goes haywire and you don't feel full after meals. Lose just a couple hours of sleep a night and you'll gain 10-15 pounds per year.

When you don't have enough sleep, you eat more and exercise less. To make matters worse, you tend to eat more unhealthy sugary foods when you're tired. Think of the last time you felt tired and groggy. Did you head to the kitchen for a bowl of broccoli?

This weight-gain puts you at risk for heart disease, diabetes, and obstructive sleep apnea (discussed below). Unfortunately, you can develop a vicious cycle of poor sleep, weight gain, obstructive sleep apnea, and then even worse sleep.

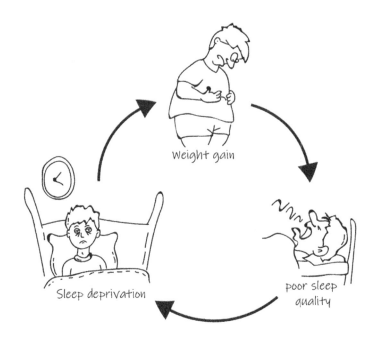

Weight gain

Sleep deprivation

poor sleep quality

The vicious cycle of sleep deprivation,
weight gain, and OSA

Infection (including COVID-19) - You're heading to the airport for a long flight and afraid of catching a cold or coronavirus on the plane. After all, you don't want to arrive in Hawaii sick or face a quarantine. Those fizzy vitamin drinks won't help you, but sleep will.

In a dramatic study where scientists sprayed the cold virus into the awaiting noses of volunteers, researchers found that folks sleeping five hours per night the week before had nearly three times the risk of developing a cold than folks sleeping seven or more hours. Sleep even improves your immune system's response to the flu vaccine. What would you do to slash your risk of suffering from a cold or flu?

This point is critical. Multiple studies show that sleep helps to protect you from respiratory viruses similar to

COVID-19. While a study hasn't been conducted specifically on sleep and COVID-19 (the coronavirus), it is highly likely that sleep deprivation will increase your chance of catching this dangerous disease.

In addition to practicing routine precautions (handwashing, distance, avoid touching your face, staying home while sick), you want to do whatever you can to boost your immune system. COVID-19 seems to inflict the most damage on the elderly and people with weak immune systems. Sleeping a full 7-8+ hours per night may be one of the very best things you can do to strengthen your immune system and protect yourself from the coronavirus.

Table 1. Tips to stay safe from the coronavirus (COVID-19 and similar viruses)

Tip	Notes
Social Distancing	• Stay at least six feet away from coughers. • Don't shake hands. Tap toes or 'bows (elbows) instead. • Avoid crowded indoor places like concerts and movie theaters. • Regular face masks probably don't help.
Seniors appear to be at greatest risk	The elderly need to be especially careful around sick people. They should avoid high-risk areas like airplanes and cruise ships.
Wash your hands frequently	Alcohol hand gel also works. Avoid touching your face, mouth, and eyes in public.
Protect other people	Stay home if you're sick. Consider calling your doctor rather than going into the office. If you're sick, please wear a mask to protect others.
Wipe down surfaces, including your phone	• Coronavirus can survive on plastic and some metal surfaces for days. • Alcohol and Clorox wipes kill coronavirus. • Wipe down your cell phone and door handles. • At work, wipe down shared computer keyboards, phones, and desks.

Air travel	• Bring a small alcohol hand gel to sanitize your hands while on the plane. • Bring wipes to clean your seatbelt, tray table, and overhead controls. • Use the overhead fan. It will blow filtered air on you and push away air from your neighbors. • Your biggest risk is from your neighbors coughing. • Don't fly if you're sick.
Sleep 7 or more hours	Sleep deprivation significantly increases your risk of illness. Keep your immune system strong and get enough sleep.
Take zinc	Zinc appears to reduce the risk of catching respiratory viruses similar to COVID-19. Take high-dose zinc for the first 5 days you have respiratory symptoms. Consider taking zinc daily as prevention (although there isn't much data on this). You're probably zinc-deficient anyway, so I advise daily zinc.
Eat garlic	Garlic boosts your immune system and seems to help protect against viruses similar to COVID-19. Aim for the equivalent of at least one clove daily.
Use probiotics	Probiotics boost your gut health and strengthen your immune system. There is evidence that they help protect people from viruses similar to COVID-19. If you take them, be sure to take a variety of organisms. Lactobacillus plantarum and Lactobacillus paracasei seem particularly beneficial. Try kombucha, sauerkraut, and kefir.

Regular, moderate exercise	Moderate exercise strengthens your immune system and appears to protect against respiratory viruses, particularly if you're already stressed.

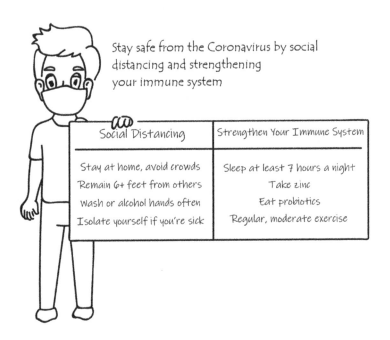

Stay safe from the Coronavirus by social distancing and strengthening your immune system

Social Distancing	Strengthen Your Immune System
Stay at home, avoid crowds	Sleep at least 7 hours a night
Remain 6+ feet from others	Take zinc
Wash or alcohol hands often	Eat probiotics
Isolate yourself if you're sick	Regular, moderate exercise

How to greet someone: tap toes or 'bows. Don't shake hands

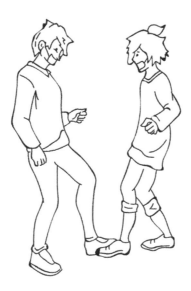

Beyond the coronavirus, adequate sleep also appears to help the immune system fight bacteria, periodontal disease, and even cancer.

Your immune system is your body's first line of defense against cancer. When abnormal cells spring up that could develop into tumors, it is your immune system's job to identify and kill these potentially troublesome cells. Mounting evidence shows that your sleep-deprived immune system is less effective at rooting out these dangerous cells, thereby making it easier for cancer to grow in your body.

To think of it another way, inadequate sleep may be considered a carcinogen.

Heart disease. The less you sleep, the more likely you'll die from a heart attack. It's that simple. And the effects add up over time.

People who sleep less than six hours per night in midlife have three times the lifetime risk of suffering from a stroke or heart attack than those who sleep at least seven hours. Think about it. That one extra hour of sleep at night can mean the difference between living a long, full life and dying early from a stroke.

Memory and learning - You have a big test tomorrow. You've been preparing for days reading and rereading your materials. This exam can mean the difference between the career of your dreams and a disappointing second choice. What should you do to maximize your chance of success with tomorrow's exam?

You guessed it. Sleep.

Sleep is one of the most powerful memory enhancement tools available. When you sleep before you study, you improve your chances of retaining the information. Ideally, you want a good night of sleep before you study. Even a nap before you start preparing for your test will help you learn and retain the information.

You also want to turn in early after you study. You'll retain 20-40 percent more information when you enjoy a good night's rest after you study for your exam. How much better will you do on the test if you remember 40% more?

Our schools start too early (a plea).

If you're a politician, school administrator, or community leader, I'd like to take this moment for a quick plea on behalf of our kids. Please start school later in the morning.

Children, particularly adolescents need extra sleep. The circadian rhythm shifts in the teenage years, causing teens to naturally fall asleep later and wake up later. Moreover, adolescents need extra sleep during their pubertal growth spurt.

But, rather than encouraging our teens to score much-needed sleep (particularly their morning REM sleep), we force them to wake up early to attend middle and high school. In essence, our school schedules are intentionally savaging our teen's life-sustaining sleep. Things are even worse for student-athletes who have early morning practice.

Unfortunately, most teens can't make up this sleep deprivation by going to bed earlier because their brains are simply not programmed to go to sleep that early (even when they're sleep-deprived). Sleeping in on the weekends won't help either since extra shuteye one day can never really make up for lost sleep on a different day.

When our teens are sleep-deprived, they're more moody and irritable. They're more impulsive and apt to make poor decisions. In fact, a lot of the obnoxious and dangerous behavior that we associate with the teenage years may be due to inadequate sleep.

Inadequate sleep causes teens to perform worse in school. They struggle to pay attention and learn new information. And, if they drive, they're more likely to have a car accident.

The good news is that we, as a society, have the power to help keep our teens out of trouble. Start school later. The American Academy of Sleep Medicine recommends that middle and high schools start at 8:30 or later.

Change is coming. To its credit, California enacted Senate Bill 328 which prevents middle schools from starting before 8 a.m. and high schools from starting before 8:30. This extra sleep will be a blessing for our kids.

If you're reading this, I beg you to please contact your school and athletic officials and lobby for later school and practice start times. Our kids need help.

Sleeping pills

Sleeping pills increase your risk of death. Research out of the University of California, San Diego revealed that folks using sleeping pills are more likely to develop cancer and succumb to all-cause mortality.

In the 2.5 year study, people using sleeping pills were nearly five times more likely to die than similar people (controls) not using the pills. The more people used the pills, the higher the risk of death. Shockingly, even infrequent users had a higher chance of dying compared to their abstaining peers. Let me repeat, if you pop even an occasional sleeping pill, you may be risking your life.

Here are some of the dangers associated with popular sleeping pills:

- Greater risk of death, even for infrequent users

- Poor-quality sleep

- Higher risk of infection, possibly due to the unnatural sleep produced by the pills

- Increased risk of cancer

- Fatal car accidents, possibly due to excessive sedation the next day

Americans pop 10 million sleeping pills per month, in the desperate hope to obtain a good night's sleep. They are fool's gold. Don't be a victim.

It's worth noting that I am not claiming that sleeping pills in principle are bad. Rather, I'm making the case that pills commonly used today are dangerous. After all, the data above was based on popular sleeping pills at the time of the studies. It is possible that one day we'll develop sleeping medications that are effective and free of dangerous side effects. I hope that day comes. Millions of people would benefit from such treatment. But, until that day arrives, there are superior options for those seeking a good night's sleep.

What about melatonin?

You've just flown from New York to Paris to conclude an important business deal. Millions of dollars and the future of your company ride on tomorrow's negotiations. Your plane lands at 11 p.m. Parisian time, but it's only 5 p.m. your (New York) time. You check into your suite at the Shangri-La Hotel, marvel at the stunning views of the Eiffel Tower, and then flip open your laptop to check your email one last time. You settle into the satiny sheets and close your eyes.

You lie there for hours, wide awake.

You toss and turn. You play soft music. You try some warm, comfy PJs, but sleep eludes you.

Is it the excitement of the trip? The anticipation of tomorrow's big meeting? Your regret over leaving your family behind in Manhattan?

Torture!

After counting sheep, thinking about your breathing, and flipping to every possible sleeping position countless times, you finally slip into blissful slumber at 5 a.m.

Your alarm howls at 7 a.m., after only two short hours of sleep. Bad news.

You walk into the meeting, tired, irritable, unfocused, and cracked out on cafés au lait. The meeting is a failure.

What should you have done differently?

It's likely that you couldn't sleep because of the time change. When you attempted to go to bed at midnight in the hotel, it was still only 6 p.m. your time. Your biological clock was primed to stay awake several more hours. It's tough to fight against biology.

It was probably a mistake to check email right before bed. The blue light from your laptop signals your brain that it's daytime, further complicating your efforts to convince yourself that it's the middle of the night. Moreover, reading emails and reviewing your meeting agenda likely created unnecessary stress. Stress is poison for sleep.

The warm PJs didn't help, either. Your body cools down as you enter the throes of sleep. In fact, a slight cooling is one of the defining features of sleep onset. It's tough to sleep in a sauna.

Finally, you could have popped a melatonin tablet.

Melatonin is a hormone produced by your brain's pineal gland. The molecule is your signal that night is approaching and it's time to wind down. Melatonin doesn't actually cause sleep. Rather, it acts as a messenger to notify the sleep circuitry in your brain that it's showtime.

Think of it this way. Parts of your brain actively cause you to sleep. But, they need to know when to kick in gear and turn on those zzzs. Melatonin alerts your sleep centers that it's bedtime.

As such, melatonin levels start to rise at dusk and peak around midnight. The hormone makes itself scarce in the morning, informing your brain that it's time to wake up.

When you tried to sleep at the Parisian hotel, your melatonin levels were low because your brain's timing centers still thought it was the late afternoon. You made matters worse with the harsh glare of your laptop.

If you took a melatonin pill two hours before your intended bedtime, you might have been able to trick your body into believing that it is time to sleep. Rather than tossing and turning, you would have been rejuvenated and ready to go for your meeting.

Jet lag is one of the few clear indications for melatonin. It helps speed up your body's adjustment to new time zones. It may benefit shift workers with inconsistent sleep times who alternate between day and night work. It might help some people with insomnia fall asleep earlier. It also appears to be helpful in the hospital, allowing patients to catch some needed rest in an otherwise noisy and scary environment.

Since melatonin is a complex hormone with a number of effects, it may also be beneficial for certain types of anxiety, high blood pressure, cancer, athletic performance, ADHD, chronic fatigue syndrome, post-surgical recovery, inflammatory bowel disease, stress, and the prevention of sunburns. The research on these diseases changes by the day, so stay tuned to see whether melatonin might help you.

If you decide to take melatonin, I suggest using 1 mg or less. There's no reason to use massive doses. Remember, our goal is to mimic your body's normal physiologic response to dusk.

One of the downsides of melatonin is the possibility of prolonged sedation. If melatonin lingers in your bloodstream, you may feel tired the next morning rather than refreshed. Therefore, I suggest testing how your body reacts.

Don't drive or do anything important the first morning after you try it. Consider experimenting with it on a weekend when you plan to sit around the house the next morning. After all, you don't want to take it for the first time and wind up in a car crash or asleep during your final exam the next day.

The other problem with melatonin is that the production of the tablets isn't regulated and quality is inconsistent. The strength of the pills may be totally different than what's on the label. Melatonin is infamous for this. Make sure you buy a reputable brand. Ideally, the pills should be tested at an independent lab. At the very least, you want the manufacturers to be GMP certified.

Summary of my advice about melatonin:

• Speak to your doctor first before starting melatonin

• It is probably most beneficial for jet lag, insomnia, and hospitalized patients

• Take 1 mg approximately two hours before your intended bedtime

- Use a reputable brand, ideally independently tested and produced at a GMP facility

- Stay home the morning after the first time you take it. You want to make sure you feel refreshed rather than hungover

- Watch out for innovative new uses for melatonin. Visit my website to keep up to date.

Obstructive sleep apnea - a thief in the night

You go to sleep every night on time. You're in bed a full eight hours. Your room is cool and dark. You don't drink coffee after breakfast and you avoid alcohol. Yet, you still feel groggy when you wake up.

You can't stay awake during meetings and your work performance suffers. Driving goes from routine to terrifying, since you doze off behind the wheel. You're losing your focus, energy, and libido.

To make matters worse, your doctor diagnoses you with high blood pressure (hypertension). She's worried about your heart and sends you to get an echocardiogram.

How did you get so sick?

The one clue comes from your wife. She tells you that you're snoring at night. Could that be the cause?

#####

If you think you have obstructive sleep apnea (OSA), you're not alone. It's estimated that 25 million adult Americans suffer from disrupted sleep due to OSA.

Here's how it works. During sleep, the muscles that hold open your airways relax a little. They sleep, too. This decreased muscle tone means that your tongue falls back, your soft palate (the fleshy tissue in the back of the throat) flops into your airways, and your breathing is just a touch less forceful. This decrease in tone is no big deal for folks without OSA. They just breathe around it.

For people with OSA, it's a different story. Their tongues and soft palate fall back and almost completely block off the airway. When someone tries to breathe around this obstruction, they snore. They gasp for air as they struggle to breathe against a blocked airway.

With mild OSA, the air struggles to reach your lungs. As OSA grows more severe, oxygen might not reach your lungs at all during periods of deep sleep. Your breathing is completely obstructed. Then, in a desperate attempt to inhale, you wake yourself up at night. When you wake up, you temporarily increase your muscle tone and take in an urgently-needed breath. Then, you fall back to sleep. You may not even realize you woke up.

Here's the pattern: snoring, respiratory pauses caused by complete airway obstruction, arousals from sleep in a desperate attempt to get air, big breath, then the return to sleep. For OSA patients, this battle for air is fought over and over throughout the night.

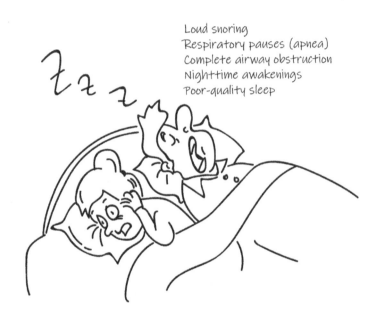

Loud snoring
Respiratory pauses (apnea)
Complete airway obstruction
Nighttime awakenings
Poor-quality sleep

Obstructive sleep apnea

All those awakenings come at a steep cost.

Here's the trouble. This cycle of airway obstruction and nighttime awakenings is like a jackhammer for your sleep. When you keep waking up, you're unable to reach and sustain the deep sleep that your body craves. It's like trying to do your taxes while a two-year-old keeps interrupting you to ask questions. It's impossible.

Your choppy sleep prevents you from maintaining rapid eye movement (REM) sleep. REM sleep is critical for creativity, communication, and emotional regulation. You're also blocked from restorative deep non-REM sleep (NREM) which is critical for health, memory, and learning.

The result is that you wake up feeling nearly as tired as you did when you went to bed. Your Swiss cheese sleep saddles you with low energy, reduced memory, diminished focus, and an impaired immune system. Poor sleep increases your risk of cancer and Alzheimer's.

Your nightly struggle for air takes a toll on your heart. People with obstructive sleep apnea are more likely to have high blood pressure, pulmonary hypertension, heart attacks, and strokes. This is serious stuff.

I really want to emphasize this point. Your nocturnal struggles for air are killing you. You can't just drink a double-shot latte and call it a day. You need to fix the sleep apnea.

Sleep study

If you have excessive daytime sleepiness, snoring, or pauses in your overnight breathing (apneas) and you're concerned you have OSA, you should see your doctor. They can evaluate you for OSA and check you for conditions associated with sleep apnea including high blood pressure (hypertension), obesity, and large tonsils.

The gold standard for diagnosing OSA is the overnight sleep study. Depending on your doctor's evaluation, it can be done either in a sleep lab or at home.

The at-home sleep test is the most common. Your doctor orders a small device that fits on a finger. It measures the oxygen level in your blood while you sleep. If you have apneas or airway obstruction, you'll pull less oxygen into your lungs and your blood oxygen levels will fall (oxygen desaturations). Your finger monitor will detect and record these desaturations. Based on their frequency and severity, your doctor can diagnose you with OSA.

Some at-home sleep tests will include additional sensors including something that fits over your face to measure the airflow and a device over your belly to measure respiratory effort. For most people, these extra sensors are not necessary to diagnose OSA.

Certain individuals might require a more formal sleep study in a laboratory. These tests include a number of extra sensors and usually have cameras that monitor your sleep. They can even use an EEG, which are wires on your head to measure your brainwaves. The EEG confirms exactly when you're asleep and can determine your sleep stage (NREM vs REM).

For the vast majority of people, the simple at-home oxygen monitor is enough to diagnose sleep apnea. It's easy and usually covered by insurance. If you suspect that you might have OSA, just go to your doctor for an evaluation and sleep study.

Let's look at some treatments for OSA.

You can test yourself

The most exciting news in sleep health is that you now have the power to test yourself for sleep apnea. There are some great devices on the market that monitor your breathing and oxygen level. They can even monitor your brain waves.

While many of these devices are not FDA approved and may not be as accurate as a sleep test you'd get from a specialist, most are quite good. I support their use because I suspect that most people lack the motivation to get off their duff go to their doctor for an exam.

You can order these devices from the comfort of your own home. They ship them to you and most are easy to use. The manufacturers will even help you interpret the results. If you have sleep apnea, your next step would then be to go to your doctor for treatment.

To be clear, I'm not suggesting that you use your own sleep test instead of going to see your doctor. I just don't want you to have OSA without realizing it. You need a diagnosis so you seek treatment. If you won't go to your doctor to get checked out, please at least go ahead and order your own test if you snore.

I order at-home sleep studies for most of my wellness patients. OSA is a common (and treatable) cause of fatigue, aging, and ill-health. Let's make sure we catch it.

Sleep Position

It turns out that the easiest treatment for OSA is one that you can start tonight.

Train yourself to sleep on your side (or stomach).

As discussed earlier, your muscle tone drops when you're asleep. When you sleep on your back, soft tissues like your tongue and tonsils flop down and block your upper airway. You struggle for air as you fight against your soft palate blocking your throat. Gravity is working against you.

Sleeping Position	Comment	
On your back	Bad news!	☹
On the right side	Ok	😐
On your stomach	Ok	😐
On the left side	Great!	☺

Sleep on your left side. For adults in the lateral position, gravity moves tissue away from your breathing passages and you breathe better. Studies show that your airways are more open on your side compared with sleeping on your back and you have fewer overnight apneas.

Interestingly, sleeping on your left side is better than the right. It might also cause you to have less acid reflux overnight.

For those unable to sleep on the left side, sleeping on your right side or stomach is still probably better than sleeping on your back. Back sleeping is to be avoided at all costs.

What to do if you are used to sleeping on your back? It turns out that there is a simple trick to train yourself to avoid your back. Sew a tennis ball or something annoying into the back of your pajama shirt. That way, you'll be uncomfortable each time you try to lie on your back. Eventually, you'll learn to sleep on your stomach. You can also buy special shirts designed to help you avoid your back.

It also helps to have the right pillow. Generally, you want a slightly firmer pillow to support your neck while lying on the side. Go ahead and try out a few side-sleeping pillows and see which is best for you.

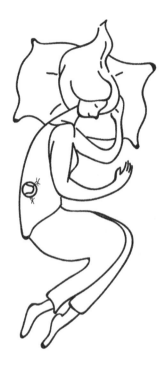

Obesity

The heavier you are, the greater the chance you'll develop OSA. Almost half of all obese adults suffer from obstructive sleep apnea. Nearly three out of four adults with OSA are obese.

By the same token, the more obese someone is, the worse their OSA.

It isn't just that obesity worsens sleep apnea. Sleep apnea contributes to obesity. People with severe OSA develop a different mix of appetite-controlling hormones which causes them to eat more and feel less satiated. Moreover, people with

OSA feel sleepier during the day and are less likely to go out and exercise.

It becomes a vicious cycle where obesity leads to OSA which leads to more obesity.

The good news is that if obese people lose even ten percent of their body weight, they can reduce or even eliminate their OSA. An overweight person with OSA should speak to their doctor about a diet and exercise program. Consider intermittent fasting. The weight loss can make the difference between a healthful night's sleep and the dreaded alternative of sleepiness, heart disease, diabetes, and stroke.

I can't emphasize this enough. If you're obese and have sleep apnea, the best thing you can do for your health is to lose weight. And, you'll find that once you start losing weight and sleeping better, it will be easier to lose more weight. You just have to get the ball rolling.

I should mention that you can have OSA even if you are not obese. It is estimated that one in four people with sleep apnea has a normal weight. Therefore, don't assume that you don't have OSA just because you're skinny. You can still have sleep apnea. That's why it's critical for all adults who snore and feel sleepy during the day to go to their doctor or sleep specialist for an exam (or order an at-home sleep study).

CPAP

CPAP, short for continuous positive airway pressure, is the leading treatment for obstructive sleep apnea in adults. For people that use it, it feels like nothing short of a miracle.

Here's how it works. You wear a soft, customized mask at night that fits over your nose and/or mouth. The mask is connected to a machine at your bedside that detects when you're breathing. The machine delivers a boost of air when you inhale and keeps your airways open when you exhale. The extra support makes it much easier to breathe at night.

With a properly-functioning CPAP device, you won't struggle for air. You'll breathe comfortably without all the nighttime awakenings and sleep disturbances.

Once you're used to the CPAP machine, your snoring will disappear. Finally, your partner will be able to sleep in the same room as you. Since you'll enjoy the benefits of quality sleep, you'll feel more refreshed in the morning. You'll have more energy, vitality, and focus. Your memory will improve and so will your mood. Note: there's more information about the importance of sleep on mood and depression in the depression chapter 6. With CPAP, you'll feel better and experience a higher quality of life.

If I haven't convinced you yet, here are some of the medical benefits of regular use of CPAP:

• Reduced risk of dying from congestive heart failure

• Decreased coronary artery disease

• Reduced risk of death from an irregular heartbeat

• Slash your risk of stroke in half

• Decreased risk of diabetes

• Smaller chance of a deadly car accident

• A happier spouse/partner/roommate

CPAP is a medical device that requires a prescription. Your sleep specialist will pick the right machine for you and adjust the settings to meet your needs. There are a variety of mask sizes and shapes, and your sleep doctor will find the right one for your face and breathing style. It may take a bit of trial and error to make it comfortable, but it will soon feel as natural as breathing.

I should note, there are tons of sleep disorders besides OSA, including insomnia, narcolepsy, sleepwalking, teeth grinding, and restless leg syndrome. I chose to focus exclusively on OSA in this chapter because it is common, causes excessive daytime sleepiness, and is easily treatable. If you're concerned that you have any kind of sleep disturbance, please go see your doctor or sleep specialist.

Sleep Hygiene - the do's and don'ts of healthy sleep

Let's end this chapter with a summary of what you should do to improve your shut-eye. These best-practices, otherwise known as sleep hygiene, are scientifically established ways you can enjoy the restorative sleep you deserve. Most of these techniques are easy to follow, and I hope you'll put them to use tonight. Share them with your friends and family and you'll be their hero.

DON'T check your email, read the news, use your cell phone, or laptop before bed. The blue light from the screens will trick your brain into thinking it's daytime and will suppress your melatonin production. In addition, most people find email and news agitating - taking you out of the relaxed state required for sleep. If you have to use electronic devices in the evening, keep the screens dim. Hold the screens as far away from your face as possible. As of this writing, it is unclear whether using a yellow tint (like the iPhone's Night Shift) will improve sleep. While it was initially thought that converting the blue light to yellow would be beneficial, the current state of research now makes this uncertain.

DO get at least seven to nine hours of sleep per night. Remember, you want a minimum of seven hours of sleep, which means you need to be in bed (with your eyes closed) more than seven hours. I would shoot for at least eight hours. And, if you think you're one of those people who only need five hours of sleep, you're wrong.

DON'T work or watch TV in your bed. You want to associate your bed with sleep and relaxation, not with stressful activities like work. If you need to work in the evening, go to a desk or your kitchen table.

DO go to sleep and wake up at the same time every day. The goal is to train your brain when it's time to go to bed.

Avoid staying up late on weekends. Bedtime is bedtime. Your brain will thank you.

DON'T have a lot of light in your bedroom. The darker the room, the easier it will be for your brain to up-cycle melatonin production. Ambient light in the room can trick your brain into thinking it's daytime. Remember, throughout nearly all of our evolution, we slept at night in the dark. Our brains weren't designed to deal with artificial lights. Some authorities recommend using red (or yellow) light in your bedroom rather than standard LED bulbs. In either case, keep your nighttime lights as dim as possible.

DO keep your bedroom cool at night. You reduce your core body temperature when you sleep. In fact, decreasing temperature is part and parcel of the sleep process. When you cool off your bedroom, you help your body enter the sleep state. Studies show improved length and quality of sleep in cool rooms. Remember, we evolved to sleep in the cooler night air. How cold should your room be? That's unclear, but probably somewhere in the mid-60s.

DON'T partake in caffeine, nicotine, alcohol, and strenuous exercise before bed. Caffeine, exercise, and nicotine are stimulants and they'll make it tougher for you to fall asleep. Unless you're highly tolerant, you should switch to decaf by the early afternoon. It can take 5-10 hours to eliminate from your body. Plan accordingly.

DO catch some rays during the day. Just as it's important to show your brain when it's night, it's equally important to train the brain for the day. Your brain needs to know day and night in order to properly set your circadian rhythm. Try to expose yourself to at least 30-60 minutes of sunlight in the morning.

DON'T eat heavy meals or drink lots of liquids close to bedtime. In particular, you want to avoid meals high in carbs, sugar, and processed foods before bed. They wreak havoc on your blood sugar levels at night and disturb your sleep. If you love dessert, enjoy it with lunch instead of dinner. If you're hungry before bed, try a piece of fruit, veggies, or a small piece of cheese. Drinking before bed might lead to frequent and disrupting trips to the restroom at night.

DO test the quality and quantity of your own sleep with wearable technology. There are some nifty devices that monitor your brainwaves and can detect OSA.

DON'T take a nap after 3 p.m. A tip from Dr. Walker. A late-afternoon nap can make it tougher to fall asleep at night. If you like naps, shoot for earlier in the day. In fact, a late-morning nap can be helpful if you anticipate missing sleep the upcoming night.

DO relax before bed. You want to put yourself in a calm mood before you lay down to sleep. Try meditation, prayer, relaxing music, or a warm bath. Everyone is different. Experiment and see what helps you unwind.

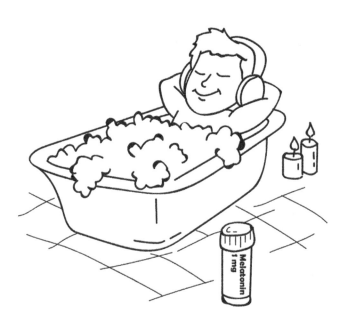

[Author's note: I realized that I wasn't practicing what I preached with sleep hygiene. While I'd keep the bedroom dark, I'd usually have the room warm and toasty. Worse, I always spent time with my cell phone before going to sleep. So, for New Years, I decided I'd keep the room below 70 and not look at my phone at night in bed except in emergencies.

I'm happy to report that so far, those small changes made a huge difference. I feel more refreshed in the morning and I don't go to the bathroom as often at night. I think my next move will be to buy an old-fashioned alarm clock to keep bedside so I don't have to look at my phone at all.]

Chapter 5

Sleep and Elite Performers

Sleep and elite athletic performance

You're on center court, sweat glistening under the intense glare of the lights. It's the final game of the final set. It's match point. You could hear a pin drop as the crowd stares at you with eager anticipation. Everyone is on the edge of their seats. The tennis ball feels cold and hard in your hands. This is it. This is the moment when champions are made.

You inhale and toss the ball in the air for your game-deciding serve.

Smash! You hit an ace. Your lightning-fast serve lands in, and just out of reach of your spent opponent. Time stops. For a moment, there is silence. Then, the crowd erupts with cheers and celebration. Today is your day, and this is your year. Congratulations, champion.

Reporters mob you after the game. What was the secret of your success? Diet? Extra practice? Different shoes?

You smile as you reveal the key to your victory.

"Sleep."

#####

This book is full of tips for high-performers and elite athletes. Of all the advice, making sure you get enough sleep is probably the most important. If you miss sleep, even for one night, your performance will suffer. Even more remarkable, if you get bonus sleep, your skills will take off like a rocket.

Unfortunately, elite athletes often suffer from sleep deprivation. Forty-two percent of college athletes reported poor sleep, with more than one in three averaging less than seven hours per night. More than half of the athletes in the study complained of excessive daytime sleepiness.

There are several reasons why sleep is critical for elite athletes. The first is that sleep helps you learn and store muscle memory. When you spend all that time refining your serve in tennis or perfecting your free throw in basketball, what you're really doing is training your brain to do a series of very complicated and delicate movements. In a way, it's just like a professional violinist practicing her concerto. The goal is to learn a precise series of actions.

But, once you learn the movements, you need to remember them.

Just as sleep helps you store explicit memories, such as the answers to your history test, sleep also helps you store muscle memory. Multiple studies prove that when you enjoy restful sleep while practicing your sport, you'll get more out of the practice. Sleep helps you improve by enhancing your muscle memory.

You don't want to waste all those practices, do you?

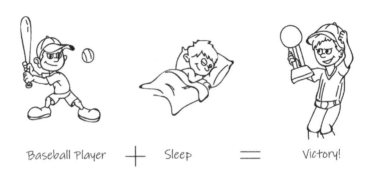

Baseball Player ━━┼━━ Sleep ══ Victory!

Secondly, sleep optimizes your body. I don't have to tell you, your body is a machine, and you want it running at peak performance. That's why you spend all that time lifting weights in the gym, running laps, and eating healthy supplements and foods. It turns out that sleep is essential to optimize your body.

Multiple studies on athletes reveal that sleep increases muscle strength, beefs up your cardiovascular system, improves your maximum jump height, shortens your reaction time, and increases your time to exhaustion.

Perhaps, most importantly, sleep deprivation increases your risk of sports injuries. Athletes averaging six hours of sleep per night were twice as likely to suffer an injury as those sleeping a full eight hours. Those sleeping nine hours suffered even fewer injuries. Think about it. If you're a professional athlete or coach, how much would you give to avoid an injury? A good night's sleep is a small price to pay for a season of health.

Finally, sleep is critical for an athlete's emotion and temperament. Well-rested athletes enjoy superior judgment, improved vigilance, enhanced alertness, and a better mood. Based on my review of the data, I suspect that tired athletes are more likely to start fights, commit fouls, and get ejected from the game.

If you're a parent, you know what it's like when your toddler is tired. All the screaming, crying, collapsing on the ground, etc. Adults are no different. You see it on the courts every day. Get some rest and you'll psychologically outlast your fatigued opponent.

Here are some of the documented harms of sleep deprivation on athletes:

• Swimmers suffer more depression, confusion, fatigue, and anger.

• Weightlifters can't bench, deadlift, or leg press as much weight. Their mood declines.

• Volleyball players are exhausted sooner.

• Tennis players have less accurate serves.

• Soccer players perform worse on sprints, kicking tests, and attention.

• Baseball players with chronic sleep deprivation have worse strike-zone judgment and shorter professional careers.

Why limit yourself to the minimum sleep necessary? The studies show that elite athletes benefit from extra sleep - above and beyond eight hours. Here are some proven benefits of sleep extension for athletes:

• Swimmers enjoy faster 15-meter sprints, reaction times of the blocks, and turn times.

• Basketball players experience faster sprints, improved shooting accuracy, and improved mood.

• Australian Football League athletes suffered less fatigue and enjoyed increased vigor.

• Tennis players benefited from more accurate serves and decreased sleepiness.

Some of the world's greatest athletes, including Roger Federer and LeBron James, are reported to sleep more than ten hours per night. If extra sleep is good enough forthem, it's good enough for you.

You're still human

You may be the greatest basketball, soccer, or sprinter of all time, but you're still a person. You're still susceptible to the same illness as everyone else.

Athletes still come down with the common cold, GI bugs, coronavirus, and the flu. Your basketball prowess won't keep the germs away. You don't want to miss practice or games because you're hacking up a lung or running to the bathroom with explosive diarrhea. *Every time you skip out on training or weightlifting because you're out sick, you're falling behind your competitors.*

Beyond colds and flu, athletes still suffer from the same medical problems as everyone else. They can get cancer, auto-immune diseases, and neurologic dysfunction. You don't want your career (or life) cut short because you sacrificed your health by skimping on sleep.

At the end of the day, the best thing you can do to improve your athletic performance is to maximize your overall health. Missing out on sleep for extra practice is misguided and will hurt your long-term health and on-field success.

Early practice

Training often starts early in the morning, particularly for student-athletes. While crack of dawn practices might make it easier to schedule other activities, they wreak havoc on your sleep.

If you start practice at 5 or 6 a.m., you'll need to wake up by 4 or 5 a.m. to arrive on time. Unless you go to bed early (around 8 p.m.), you won't sleep your full eight hours. Since most people go to bed considerably later, you'll only bank a paltry 5-6 hours of sleep. As we discussed earlier in the chapter, this sleep deprivation will slow you down, harm your mood, impair your reflexes, and diminish your shot accuracy.

Worst of all, it will make you more likely to suffer an injury. Depending on your bedtime, your 6 a.m. practice might literally double your chance of injury compared to an 8 a.m. practice.

As a coach, you have real power to improve the health and performance of your players simply by rescheduling practices slightly later in the day. It's a much easier fix than other performance-enhancing options. If you're unable to reschedule practice, find a way to enforce an earlier bedtime for your athletes. Don't let them stay up late tweeting.

The other problem with early practices is that they disproportionately devastate REM sleep. Here's the deal. We sleep in cycles, collecting bits of NREM and REM sleep throughout the night. However, we score most of our deep NREM sleep in the early part of the night and we bank most of our dreamy REM sleep in the last few hours of our slumber.

If you have an early-morning practice, it is likely that you're missing a large chunk of your critical REM sleep. It's a big loss. REM sleep is responsible for improving creativity, comprehension, and decision-making skills. Chop off REM sleep, and you'll lose judgment. Your ability to "read the minds" of your opponents will be impaired and your team communication will suffer.

Night games

Shift-work is tough on the body. Sleep loss and irregular sleep times can increase the risk of diabetes, stroke, car accidents, death, and Alzheimer's disease.

While night games do not require staying up all night, the research shows that football players typically sleep 2-3 hours less after a night game compared with a normal night. When you consider that these athletes are probably not getting enough sleep at baseline, the loss of 2-3 hours is serious. Assuming they drive home safely, practice the next day will be impaired and health will suffer.

As a coach or player, you likely have no control over overnight games. Fortunately, however, you still have several options to minimize their harmful impact. Here are a few tips I give when I consult with coaches and elite athletes:

- Schedule naps before the night game. Ideally, the nap should be earlier in the day (between 10 a.m. and 1 p.m.) and should last for 90-120 minutes. While naps won't completely eliminate the harm from the late game, they will restore some lost sleep and will increase alertness and focus during the game.

- If you're traveling to the game, build your travel plans to allow for an appropriate period of sleep before and after the game.

- Adjust your training schedule before and after the game so that your players have enough time in bed. Don't hit them with an early workout the day of (or the day after) the game. Let them recover.

- Lobby your athletic organizations to play night games as early in the evening as possible. Your voice can make a difference. In 2019, Major League Baseball (MLB) moved their Sunday night games one hour earlier.

- Practice the sleep hygiene habits mentioned in the previous chapter. In particular, avoid alcohol and caffeine later in the day. Sleep in a cool, dark, room. And no unnecessary cell phone use before bed.

Travel and jet lag

Teams with excessive travel pay a price. The sleep deprivation caused by long travel, along with the associated jet lag from time-zone changes, harm health and degrade performance.

Major League Baseball is known for frequent travel. A study found that MLB teams crossing more than one time zone experienced significant jet lag and performed worse on the field. Recognizing the harmful consequences of jet lag, the National Hockey League (NHL) reconfigured its conferences in 2013 to decrease the need for long-distance travel.

We discussed jet lag in more detail in the previous chapter. Here are a few pieces of advice I give to my elite athlete clients:

• On the morning of your arrival, go in the sun for 30-60 minutes to help reset your circadian clock.

• If you're traveling east, go to bed early. Try to go to sleep at the proper time for your new time zone. This means avoiding caffeine, alcohol, blue light (cell phones and computers), and late practices before bedtime.

• Avoid high-carbohydrate dinners and late-night snacks.

• Consider 1 mg of high-quality melatonin about 2 hours before bedtime in the new time zone. Be sure to test your reaction to melatonin in an unimportant setting first. You may want to skip out on the melatonin if your game is early the next morning.

• Arrive at your destination early enough to allow for proper sleep.

Struggling for air after retirement

For some athletes, retirement isn't the end of their sleep woes. A study of retired football players revealed some scary results. According to this report, over half the retired NFL players suffered from sleep-disordered breathing (SDB), a close cousin of sleep apnea. In other words, more than one in two former football stars is gasping for air overnight.

The story is even worse for linemen (offensive and defensive). They have even higher rates of SDB than other players. Beyond the sleep-disordered breathing, the lineman are saddled with astronomically high rates of high blood pressure (hypertension).

These stark findings mean that former football players, particularly lineman, are at high risk for cardiovascular disease.

While the causes of these problems aren't entirely clear, the SDB and hypertension are likely related to obesity. It's not uncommon for some former athletes to gain weight due to poor diet and decreased exercise compared with their days on the gridiron.

I suspect that the risk of SDB and hypertension aren't limited to former football players and weightlifters. Any former athlete who gains weight and decreases his or her exercise regimen is probably at risk for nighttime sleep disorders and poor cardiovascular health with age.

I would advise all former athletes, particularly those on the heavier side, to go and get tested for sleep apnea and high blood pressure. The tests are easy and they might just save your life.

Even though you may be an elite performer, you may still have depression. In the next chapter, we'll review how to diagnose and treat depression. Read on.

Chapter 6

Depression and the Ketamine Revolution

The sun rises, but you can't climb out of bed. The day holds no interest to you.

You no longer enjoy your job. The work feels meaningless.

Food, once one of your great joys, lost its appeal. You no longer eat to live, you live to eat. And probably not as much as you should. You're losing weight.

You feel less motivated at work and in life. Hopelessness, fatigue, and disinterest replace your formerly vibrant self. Pessimism reigns.

Even your friends and family, the loves of your life, can't lift your spirits. Where did your happiness go?

Consider another example. You're a professional basketball player. You're good enough to remain on the team, but you feel like your best days are behind you. You don't want to show up for practice. When you're playing, you feel like you're just going through the motions. There is little joy in victory. The court, the game, the fans, the win—they mean nothing.

After the game, you drive home in your expensive sports car. It's red, fast, and feels utterly pointless. You don't want to go out with your friends to celebrate. Why bother?

You unlock your door and curl up on the couch. You ask yourself, are you a fraud? Do you deserve to be out there on the court? When will everyone realize how terrible you are?

You look at the bottle of vodka in the kitchen. Is that the answer? You pour yourself a glass, hoping it will numb the pain.

These are stories of depression.

Sadly, millions of Americans and people across the globe suffer from this silent thief. It robs you of your drive, happiness, and energy. It steals the pleasure from your favorite tasks and leaves you with doubt and apathy.

I call it the silent thief because depression is often missed or misdiagnosed. You can't see depression and it doesn't show up on an X-ray or CT scan. There is no blood test. The symptoms are often vague and the presentation varies from person to person. Some depressed people barely eat, while others eat too much. Some don't sleep, while others sleep for 16 hours a day. While everyone with depression suffers, each person suffers in their own way.

Friends often misread depression. They may downplay it in the hopes of cheering you up. Even those closest to you will say that it's all in your head. They tell you that you just need to get back on your feet. They'll tell you to take a vacation, go on a date, or find a new job. These folks mean well, but their advice won't work.

That's part of depression's cruelty. Diagnosis is tough and treatment is even tougher. Many of our current medications don't work well for most people. While Prozac, Zoloft, or Paxil might lift the dark fog of depression for some, there are many who are left behind with nothing but side effects and self-doubt.

In this chapter, we'll take a look at some of the signs of depression and how we currently treat the disease. Then, we'll discuss a radically new and effective cure for depression: the Ketamine Revolution.

Symptoms of depression

Before we continue, I must say that clinical depression is a serious illness. If you suspect that you or a loved one has depression, I strongly suggest that you contact your doctor or mental health professional. While I am a doctor, I am not your doctor. If you suspect you have depression, you need to speak to a trained expert in-person who can help you. If you feel you have a psychological emergency, you should call 911 for immediate help. The Substance Abuse and Mental Health Services Administration (SAMHSA) has a government-run 24-hour helpline and they can be reached at 1-800-622-HELP. This book is not meant to be a substitute for an in-person visit with a medical professional.

Now, with that important note out of the way, what is depression? Below are the most common symptoms of depression:

• Loss of energy

• Suicidal thoughts

• Loss of interest in formerly enjoyable activities (anhedonia)

• Feeling sad or empty much of the day

• Lack of motivation - difficulty getting out of bed in the morning or giving up on work or school

• Hopelessness - the feeling that things won't get better

• Sleep disturbances - sleeping too much or too little, insomnia

• Feelings of worthlessness, guilt, or shame

- Chronic pain without a clear cause - for example, recurrent abdominal pain without a medical source of the pain

- Irritability and frequent lashing out

- Loss of focus and difficulty remembering things

- Eating disturbances - not eating enough or eating too much (in contrast to how someone ate before they were depressed)

It's important to note that the mental health disease of depression is different than feeling depressed about an event or individual external experience. We all have transient feelings of sadness and hopelessness with tragic events like divorce or the loss of a loved one. We might even experience sleep and eating disturbances. The key, however, is that these feelings are easily explained and temporary. After a period of grief, they go away.

Clinical depression is different. Folks with the disease of depression have many of the above symptoms most of the time for a prolonged period. In addition, a doctor must rule out other diseases that might masquerade as depression including substance abuse, seasonal affective disorder, hormone abnormalities, and bipolar disorder.

I'm rich, can I have depression?

Wait a minute, you may be thinking. You've got a great career as a successful CEO/doctor/lawyer/athlete/politician. Can you possibly have depression?

The answer is a resounding yes.

Depression doesn't just mean that you're in bed all day. Plenty of successful people suffer from depression. Millions do. Lots of successful folks struggle with feelings of emptiness.

Someone can be a prosperous business person and still be riddled with self-doubt, anxiety, anhedonia, and thoughts of suicide. You may be at the top of your game, yet take little pleasure in your achievements.

A lot of successful people struggled with the darkness of depression. Musicians Lady Gaga and Katy Perry, Olympian Michael Phelps, actress Gwyneth Paltrow, author J.K. Rowling, football legend Terry Bradshaw, and astronaut Buzz Aldrin were all reported to have suffered from depression. As you can see, depression spares no profession.

You may be a top executive, well-to-do attorney, or elite baseball player and still be depressed.

I urge you to speak with your doctor or mental health professional if you feel you might be depressed, even if you are a professional success. Life can get better for you. Even your career can improve.

Depression is a terrible disease that we all need to take seriously. Depression debilitates millions of Americans, impacting rich and poor alike. The trouble is, most of our treatment options are not very effective.

Depression and aging

We cannot separate the mind from the body, we're one whole. When the mind struggles, so does the body. Such is the case with depression. There is some data that depression alters your cells and actually ages you from the inside.

As discussed throughout the book, telomere length is considered a marker for cellular aging. As a rough approximation, the shorter the telomeres, the "older" the cell.

According to multiple studies, people with depression have shorter telomeres.

Depression is associated with shorter telomeres throughout the body. Telomeres were particularly short in people with the most severe depression and in people who were depressed for the longest time.

While the cause of the depression-telomere relationship is unclear at this time, some researchers believe that depression causes inflammation. As you know, inflammation is a major driver of aging. Although we don't yet have enough data to definitively say whether treating depression will lengthen telomeres, I can say that treated depression is better for your body than untreated depression.

Today's approaches to treatment aren't great

The mainstay of depression treatment is medication. The most commonly used drugs are called selective serotonin reuptake inhibitors (SSRIs) like Zoloft, Prozac, Paxil, and Celexa. These medications are and should be the initial treatment for most people. If those treatments fail, doctors might try other medications that work slightly differently, like Effexor, Cymbalta, Pamelor, and Wellbutrin.

Table 1. Problems with antidepressants

Problem	Description
Poor efficacy	Many people don't improve. Those that do improve often experience only a slight change in their symptoms.
Side effects	Even the most popular medications have significant side effects, including sexual dysfunction and weight gain. Many oral antidepressants cause dry mouth, which can lead to periodontal disease and aging.
They require a long-term commitment	Antidepressant pills don't cure depression, they manage it. They aren't like an antibiotic that you take for a week to kill off the bad germs. You may need to take them every day for the rest of your life.
Huge societal cost	As mentioned, we spend over $14 BILLION per year on these medicines. Based on the history of drug prices, these costs will likely continue to increase.

So, what to do if you suffer from depression but antidepressant pills don't work for you or you can't tolerate the side effects? Most psychiatrists will recommend trying a different class of antidepressant pills and experimenting with psychological interventions like cognitive behavioral therapy (CBT).

For severe cases of depression that don't respond to conventional treatment, psychiatrists will try electroconvulsive therapy (ECT). ECT shocks the anesthetized patient's brain with a burst of electricity. The goal is to induce a brief, controlled, generalized seizure. Depending on the protocol, the treatment is repeated several times a week for a total of 6-12 sessions.

ECT is highly-effective for many patients with severe depression. It can sometimes work even when other treatments like SSRIs have failed.

After the patient has a morning fast, the anesthesiologist will then induce general anesthesia. Then, the psychiatrist administers a carefully calibrated shock to trigger the seizure. The patient wakes up in the recovery room and goes home.

The most common adverse effects of ECT are confusion, memory loss, and the risks from general anesthesia. It is a major medical procedure with lots of uncertainty.

There's no doubt that ECT can be a life-saver for some people with treatment-resistant severe depression. For those who fail CBT and multiple antidepressants, ECT might be the only path for a new life free of anxiety, doubt, and sadness.

Or, is it?

The Ketamine Revolution

What if I told you that there is a powerful, new way to wash away the storm clouds of depression?

It's not a pill

You don't take it every day—or even every week.

There is no sexual dysfunction and or weight gain. It doesn't have the side effects of the other antidepressants.

You don't have to worry about shocking your brain or the risks of general anesthesia that you have to deal with when you have ECT.

Best of all, it works for lots of people, even folks who didn't get better with other treatments and medications. It can even help people who failed ECT.

Ketamine is different from the other treatments for depression. It's easier to take and appears to be more effective.

Here's how it works. You need to first be evaluated by a trained physician to make sure that you're a candidate for ketamine. Most doctors will recommend that you try at least one other antidepressant before starting ketamine.

Once you're approved for ketamine treatment, you'll be booked for an appointment at an office or specialty clinic. They'll place an IV and give you an infusion over 30-60 minutes. Typically, you'll relax in the office for a bit after treatment and then head home.

Remarkably, some people enjoy dramatic improvements in their depression from just one treatment. In one study published in the prestigious JAMA Psychiatry, nearly three out of every four depressed patients treated with ketamine improved after their first dose. For many, their depression was cured.

Even more impressive, many people felt better in only two hours. Two hours! Imagine that. In less than the amount of time it takes to watch Star Wars, your depression might be treated forever.

It is true that the majority of people will need several ketamine treatments to maintain a normal mood. Some doctors will administer the medicine six or more times to achieve an optimal response. Other doctors will give occasional ketamine maintenance treatments every few months in order to continue treatment success.

155

The treatment must be tailored to the individual patient. That's why it's critical that anyone considering ketamine treatment for depression goes to a physician who is an expert in the use of ketamine. Since the use of ketamine for depression is only a few years old, most people don't have the experience level required to use ketamine correctly.

For example, there are many different ways to administer ketamine. As we discussed, the most studied way to use ketamine is through an IV. But, it can also be administered from a nasal spray, orally, an injection just under the skin, or an injection into the muscle (like a vaccine). We're still working out the optimal dose and frequency of the ketamine treatment. You'll want to work with an expert who can monitor you for side effects.

Fortunately, side effects from standard doses of ketamine for depression are mild. The most common are temporary changes in heart rate and blood pressure. Some people might experience transient confusion, hallucinations, or disorientation. Thankfully, these are usually well-tolerated and go away on their own.

Is ketamine right for you?

While anesthesiologists have been using ketamine in the operating room for 50 years, it's a relative newcomer to the treatment of depression. The early studies are very promising, but we don't have nearly as much experience with ketamine as an antidepressant as we do for some other medications like Prozac.

Therefore, I agree with other experts that a depressed patient should try using a more conventional antidepressant before turning to ketamine. I say that only because there is more long-term experience with those drugs.

Having said that, I think there is clear and compelling evidence that ketamine should be tried in most people who don't improve with another medicine.

I recently interviewed the founder of the ketamine program at a major California medical center. Their policy is to use ketamine only on people who have failed other therapies (treatment-resistant depression). His patients were the toughest of the tough to treat. To our amazement, he was able to treat more than half of these challenging patients with ketamine; a remarkable success.

Ketamine gave a lifeline to people with a disease that nothing else could cure. Now, these folks can go and enjoy time with their families, return to work, and find joy in life. Many had given up hope, and now they are back on their feet with new optimism.

Imagine it. People who couldn't get out of bed in the morning are now taking their grandkids out for ice cream. People who looked in the mirror and saw only failure are now dressed up and ready for job interviews. It feels like the sunlight returned to wash away the darkness. I suspect that there are a lot more people who will benefit from ketamine. Men who suffer alone with sexual dysfunction from their antidepressant pills. Women who won't apply for a job because they are overwhelmed with hopelessness and feelings of inadequacy. Seniors who have given up, who feel their best days are behind them.

For many people, ketamine may be the answer.

If you experienced the symptoms of depression for more than a few weeks, I urge you to make an appointment with your physician or mental health professional. Even if you've failed treatment with other medications, ask them whether ketamine might be right for you.

If you do decide to seek ketamine therapy, be sure you go to someone who understands the medicine and how to use it. Since science changes by the day, you want someone who is on top of the latest research.

Other benefits of ketamine

A young girl with cancer came to me in tears. It was her leg. She was debilitated by severe pain and it was worsening by the day. The pain prevented her from walking and sleeping. Her doctors (all of them excellent) tried treatment after treatment for her pain. Pills, fentanyl, diet, therapy. Nothing made much of a difference.

We decided to treat her with an intensive ketamine infusion. By the next day, her tears vanished and she was smiling again. While not cured, she felt so much better, she was finally able to sleep. She could participate in physical therapy and even have some fun with the other kids in the hospital's playroom.

Ketamine is much more than an antidepressant. I routinely use it for my patients to both treat and prevent pain. It's such a remarkable drug, if you give it to someone before surgery, they'll have less pain after surgery—even days later. We use ketamine in the operating room to decrease or eliminate the need for dangerous narcotics.

Ketamine can successfully treat or improve a variety of pain conditions including post-surgical pain, neuropathic pain, pain from traumatic spinal cord injury, complex regional pain syndrome (CRPS), and severe headaches. Ketamine might be particularly beneficial for people with both pain and depression.

Due to ketamine's success in treating people who suffer from depression with anxious features, we've started using ketamine to treat severe anxiety. New research suggests that ketamine is an effective treatment for social anxiety disorder. Ketamine can also help people with post-traumatic stress disorder (PTSD) and obsessive-compulsive disorder.

Non-medical treatments for depression: diet, cognitive behavioral therapy, and sleep

Drugs aren't the only answer to depression. There are some simple steps that you can take right now that can improve your mood and fight this dangerous disease.

Healthy food can be enough to improve depression, according to a remarkable study published in 2019. Because this is so dramatic and so easy to do at home, I want to share the details with you.

They looked at depressed young adults and asked them to change their eating habits. Here's what they had to eat:

• Five servings of veggies per day

• Two to three servings of fruit per day

• Three servings of whole grains per day

• Three servings of protein per day (tofu, lean meat, eggs, beans)

• Three servings of unsweetened dairy per day

• Three tablespoons of nuts per day

• Two tablespoons of olive oil per day

• Three servings of fish per week

• Healthy spices like turmeric and cinnamon most days

• And they were asked to reduce the consumption of sugar, refined carbs, fatty meat, and soda

In essence, they asked the study subjects to adopt the Mediterranean diet.

Here's what happened. In just three weeks, participants significantly reduced their symptoms of depression. The improvement was so dramatic that based on a commonly-used depression scale (CESD-R score), the average person in the diet group cured their depression. And the benefits didn't

159

stop there. The healthy diet group cut their anxiety scores in half.

Think about it. This powerful, randomized, controlled study demonstrated that a healthy diet filled with veggies, nuts, fish, turmeric, and minimal sugar can help treat both depression and anxiety.

Why wouldn't you try it?

If you'd like to give this healthy, depression-fighting diet a try, here are the key takeaways. Eat as many veggies as you can. Add olive oil to your food. Eat fish several times a week. Use turmeric and other healthy spices like cinnamon and oregano as much as possible. And, perhaps most importantly, minimize sugar. These eating tips will boost your mood and overall vitality.

People with depression, particularly severe depression, often have low zinc levels. While the reason for this is unclear, it may be due to inflammation. Since zinc is such a critical mineral for regulating health and brain function, I check zinc levels on all of my patients. Zinc supplementation can improve the performance of other antidepressants. If you have depression, I suggest you ask your psychiatrist or wellness consultant whether you should test your zinc levels and take extra as a supplement.

Cognitive-behavioral therapy (CBT) is a structured form of psychotherapy that helps you reframe how you look at situations. The goal is to become aware of inaccurate or negative thinking so you can respond more constructively to challenges. There are often four steps in CBT: identify difficult situations in your life, become aware of your emotions and thoughts, identify inaccurate or negative thinking, reframe or transform your negative thoughts. Unlike some forms of psychotherapy, CBT focuses on current emotions and thoughts rather than on childhood incidents.

CBT appears to be modestly effective for depression. It can be used alone or in combination with medication like ketamine or oral antidepressants. One thing I like about CBT is that it appears to have benefits across the age spectrum. Research supports its use for adolescents and the elderly. It may be worth trying CBT for younger and elderly people with depression, people who might otherwise not be good candidates for drug therapy.

Obstructive Sleep Apnea

People with depression often have disordered sleep. For years, it was thought that depression caused sleep disturbances. Now, it appears that poor sleep contributes to depression. The worse your sleep, the more likely you'll suffer from depression.

This is good news.

Since abnormal sleep contributes to depression, that means that we can help prevent or treat depression by improving sleep quality and quantity. Sleep gives us an easy target to improve your mood.

If you snore, you might have a serious medical condition called obstructive sleep apnea (OSA). OSA is caused when your airways are partly blocked while sleeping, making breathing difficult. You struggle for air and you suffer from low blood oxygen levels.

In a desperate attempt to get air, your body will wake up over and over to force you to take a deep breath. Your sleep quality is poor and you don't enjoy the restorative benefits of quality sleep. You wake up feeling tired and groggy in the morning.

Your nighttime battles for air wreak havoc on your daytime mood.

How to improve depression without drugs
Non-pharmacologic techniques to improve depression

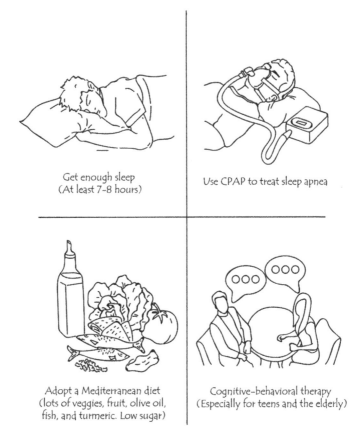

Get enough sleep
(At least 7-8 hours)

Use CPAP to treat sleep apnea

Adopt a Mediterranean diet
(lots of veggies, fruit, olive oil,
fish, and turmeric. Low sugar)

Cognitive-behavioral therapy
(Especially for teens and the elderly)

Thankfully, there is a device that will treat your OSA and improve the quality of your nighttime sleep. A CPAP machine feeds you extra air at night and helps stent open your breathing passages. It can reduce or eliminate your OSA and improve the quality of your sleep.

WHY DOCTORS SKIP BREAKFAST

It is also a powerful antidepressant.

CPAP reduces the symptoms of depression in nearly 100% of people with both depression and OSA, according to a study published in the prestigious Journal of Clinical Sleep Medicine. Think about it, nearly every single person benefitted from CPAP. There are hardly any medicines out there that boast that kind of result. It is far more successful than antidepressants.

Speaking of antidepressants, about one-third of the depressed patients were able to stop their antidepressants after starting CPAP. I don't know about you, but I'd rather use a machine to improve the quality of my breathing than take pills that mask the symptoms of poor sleep.

Depression and quarantine

Social distancing is particularly hard on people with depression. Isolation forcefully separates the depressed from their support systems. They may be unable to spend time with friends, relatives, and therapists. To make matters worse, isolation might prevent people with depression from participating in uplifting activities like athletics, enjoying a nice meal, or playing with children.

Isolation can be psychologically toxic even for people without preexisting depression. In a study of Canadians isolated for SARS, nearly a third of people developed PTSD or depressive symptoms from the separation.

If you know someone with depression who is socially isolated, please reach out to them. Call them, video chat, or send them a care package. Show them that you're there to help. Support them, even if you're separated by distance. We must all come together as a community.

If you are depressed, contact your mental health professional. Many offer phone on online visits. Teletherapy is increasingly common and can help those in need.

Summary

If you think you have depression, you're not alone. Depression is a silent, crippling disease that can rob you of your energy, hope, and joy. It's often explained away by friends ("you just have the blues, you'll be fine tomorrow") and misdiagnosed by doctors.

Unfortunately, depression's harmful effects are very real. Sufferers often withdraw from social situations, struggle to maintain relationships, underperform at work, and take little pleasure in their favorite hobbies. It is especially tough to diagnose depression because it's different for every sufferer. There is no blood test. Some depressed people can't climb out of bed in the morning while others have prestigious careers. Don't assume that your success on the field or in the boardroom means you don't have depression. It can strike anyone.

If you suspect that you may be depressed, you should speak with a doctor or mental health expert. Try to improve your diet by eating more fish, veggies, olive oil, and turmeric. Cut out the sugar. Make sure you're getting enough sleep and speak to your doctor about an overnight evaluation for obstructive sleep apnea, especially if you snore. Consider cognitive behavioral therapy.

After that, your next step is to try an antidepressant. While they offer little benefit for many people, they're fantastic for others. You won't know whether you're responsive to them until you try.

If all these treatments fail, you might be a candidate for ketamine therapy or ECT. In the right hands, ketamine treatment is remarkably successful and might offer you a long-term cure.

Depression is a treatable disease. The good news is that therapies are improving by the day and hope is on the horizon.

Get help. Don't suffer in silence.

Chapter 7:

Putting It All Together

We have control over our health and happiness.

We don't have to sit back and wait for old age to claim us. We don't have to suffer through sleepless nights and unproductive days. And we no longer need to battle depression with weak, daily medications loaded with side effects.

Thanks to modern wellness we can look forward to more dinner with friends and family, more trips to the park with our kids and grandkids, more time playing with your dog, more vacations, more books, more movies, more wins, and more celebrations.

Thanks to extra healthy years, we enjoy the zest and energy of youth while preserving our wisdom and experience.

What will you do with your extra healthspan? Will you start a new career, learn a second (or third?) language, travel the world with your spouse, start a business with your daughter, or volunteer to help disadvantaged kids? Maybe you'll pick up a new hobby (or ten). Why not learn French cuisine, oil painting, baseball, or law?

With an extra 5, 10, or even 20 healthy and energetic years, the world is your oyster.

#####

Years ago, I moved into a home in the hills near Berkeley, California. I met the former owner over lunch and he shared his story. It haunts me to this day.

Three years earlier, two married couples and long-time friends hatched a beautiful retirement plan. They bought homes right next to each other and pitched in to buy an RV. Together, the four of them would spend their golden years in each other's company. They'd grow old together, sipping glasses of wine while enjoying the sunset over the hills. On weekends, they'd play cards over breakfast or visit the local farmer's market. They'd jump in the RV for and travel through state parks and small towns, enjoying one adventure after the next. Everything was set for a dream retirement.

And it was a dream... for a year. After that one magical year of adventure and excitement, the wheels started to fall off. Age came for them. One of the four died early from heart disease. Another developed Parkinson's, with terrible shaking and an inability to care for himself. The third suffered from rapid-onset Alzheimer's dementia requiring a nursing home. And the fourth had to move back in with his adult kids in Los Angeles, taking only a suitcase of clothes and shreds of a retirement foreclosed.

Their story lived in the walls and DNA of my new home. They were with me, those wonderful retirees with their romantic dreams unfulfilled. That story, those four unfortunate souls, and my home in the hills shaped who I am today. From their experience, I learned two important lessons.

First, don't put all your dreams off until retirement. Our future is never guaranteed, despite our best plans. Second, we should do everything we can to preserve our health and vitality well into our senior years.

Based on monumental research, I am now convinced that we have a choice. We can take action now to exponentially improve our odds of enjoying a robust and vibrant retirement. We can take action now to improve our mood and kick depression to the curb. And we can take action now to make sure that we're here for our kids, grandkids, and great-grandkids.

The best part is that we don't have to wait 20 or 30 years to benefit from healthy lifestyle choices. If we do the right things now for our health, we'll have more energy for our kids, enhanced performance on the athletic field, and sharply improved productivity at work. We'll be better parents, siblings, managers, leaders, and friends.

I've reviewed hundreds of books and research papers and interviewed some of the world's leading experts. I then took my physician's critical eye to the data and sorted the good stuff from the fluff. I discarded the poorly-done studies and zeroed in on the tips and techniques that will have value for you and your family.

Here is my summary of best practices to improve your longevity and healthspan. With complete transparency, I divided my recommendations into three categories:

Strong recommendations - While new research comes out all the time, there is substantial evidence to support doing all the items on this list. All the recommendations on this list are either backed up by strong scientific research or they have fairly strong support and minimal to no side effects, meaning that they appear to be safe. Their advantages far outweigh their disadvantages.

Moderate recommendations - This is some cutting-edge stuff. All the items on this list are likely to help you live a longer, healthier life. But, the items on this list either have less evidence proving their benefits or they have a greater risk of side effects. Having said that, I still recommend implementing all the items here. As good body hackers, we'll keep our eyes open for new research.

Don't do - All the items here are clearly harmful. They'll deal a body blow to your health and they'll age you. Stay away from these bad seeds as best as you can.

Strong Recommendations:

- Skip breakfast.

- Sleep at least 7-8 hours per night. That doesn't mean 7-8 hours in bed, I mean at least 7 hours of actual sleep. Some people need even more.

- If you sleep at least 7-8 hours per night, you may be less likely to suffer from the coronavirus and other respiratory viruses. A sleep-deprived society is at greater risk for infections and pandemics.

- Get tested for obstructive sleep apnea if you snore and you're sleepy during the day. See a doctor or order a reputable home sleep apnea test device.

- Use a CPAP machine and sleep on your left side if you have OSA.

- Practice sleep hygiene. Sleep in a cool, dark room, avoid alcohol and caffeine later in the day, don't exercise right before bed, avoid electronics like phones right before sleep, and go to sleep the same time each day. If you use your phone before bed, hold it as far from your face as possible.

- Catch some morning sunlight. It will help maintain your circadian rhythm, boost your vitamin D levels, and improve your mood. Early-morning light is less harmful to your skin (lower UV index) and you may not need sunscreen.

- Avoid bright room light, particularly blue LED light, before bed. Dim your bedroom lights and replace some of your bulbs with red or yellow.

- If you feel depressed, suicidal, or hopeless, go speak to a mental health professional to be evaluated for depression. Warning signs include excessive anxiety, loss of interest in formerly pleasurable activities, and disturbed sleep and eating habits. Remember, you can hold down a successful job and still have depression.

- If you have depression, try cognitive behavioral therapy and/or an oral antidepressant. Follow the other recommendations on this list, as many of them are proven to help relieve depression. A healthy Mediterranean diet may improve your depression.

- If your depression doesn't improve with an oral antidepressant, speak to an expert about ketamine treatment.

- Athletes and coaches should work to minimize early morning practices, night games, and unnecessary travel across time zones.

- Drink coffee, preferably unsweetened. You'll live longer, protect your brain, and ward off aging with the brew's rich blend of antioxidants. You can probably safely have up to around 5 cups a day. Stop drinking caffeinated beverages sometime between 11 a.m. and 3 p.m. so as not to disrupt your sleep.

- Use continuous glucose monitoring along with a dietary journal. Create a personalized meal plan that works best for your body.

- Take resveratrol (1000 mg) and/or pterostilbene (150 mg) daily.

- In conjunction with your wellness physician, check your labs. In particular, be sure you're tested for:

  ○ Fasting insulin and glucose

  ○ Hemoglobin A1c

  ○ Testosterone level (for men)

  ○ Homocysteine

  ○ Zinc levels

  ○ TTG and DGP to evaluate for gluten sensitivity

  ○ ESR and CRP to measure inflammation

- Minimize radiation exposure. Avoid unnecessary medical tests. Ask your doctor if you can have an MRI or ultrasound instead of a CT scan.

- Eat as many veggies, herbs, and spices as you can, preferably organic. They're packed with anti-aging compounds and they're delicious. Shoot for at least 5 servings of veggies a day and as many herbs as your palate will tolerate. Some of the healthiest herbs are oregano, mustard (mixed with cruciferous veggies), marjoram, garlic, and turmeric. Enjoy dark chocolate not processed with alkali.

- Eat at least three servings of fatty fish (like wild salmon, mackerel, and sardines) a week. Eat walnuts, chia seeds, and seaweed regularly.

- Liberally use olive and walnut oils. Try them raw on salad, tomatoes, or sourdough bread.

- Minimize your sugar intake. If you want dessert, go for whole fruit or dark chocolate.

- Your mother was right, stress is bad news. It shortens your telomeres and ages you. Whenever possible, remove yourself from stressful situations and learn positive stress management techniques like meditation (see below), breathing, and exercise. Consider meeting with a therapist, adopting a pet, and trying a float tank. If you're in a highly stressful or dangerous relationship, seek immediate help.

- Regularly practice meditation, mindfulness, gratitude, breathwork, tai chi, qigong, and yoga. Be kind to others. Be there to support your friends, family, and those in need. You'll reduce your stress, decrease inflammation, boost your work performance, and lengthen your telomeres.

- Spend time with friends and family. Strong social connections keep you young and happy. Remember your parents and grandparents. Visit them as much as you can.

- Exercise regularly. Aim for at least 45 minutes of moderate+ aerobic exercise at least three times a week. Be sure to include resistance (weight) training. Exercise is anti-aging, fights almost all major diseases, decreases your risk of falls, and will increase your energy level. Plus, it lengthens your telomeres.

• Get your home tested for radon. It is a killer (and will age you). Tests are easy and inexpensive. In fact, there's a kit available from Amazon that's only $15 and you can get it delivered the next day. Do it.

• If you have pain, consider trying out a TENS unit. It is particularly effective for back, neck, bone, joint, labor, and cancer pain. Give it a shot. It's inexpensive and safe.

• Take care of your dental health. Brush and floss regularly. Use mouthwash. Visit your dentist at least twice a year. And, avoid eating sugar. Decreased oral inflammation will reduce inflammation throughout your body and prevent aging.

Moderate Recommendations:

• Sleep extra before major events like big tests or athletic competitions. Supplementary sleep appears to boost performance.

• Replace blue light with yellow hues before bedtime on your phone and computer. It is likely that the yellow color is less stimulating than the blue, although the jury is still out on this topic. Most phones and computers allow you to make the switch.

• Use high-quality, independently-tested melatonin to treat jet lag, insomnia, and sleep deprivation while in the hospital. Elite athletes may want to use low-dose melatonin an hour or two before bed when they travel multiple time zones for a game, but you should first test your body's reaction to it on an off day.

• Take metformin (between 850-1000 mg) at least several times a week. It will help keep you young.

• Consider testing yourself for ApoE4. You can have zero, one, or two copies of this gene. The more copies you have, the greater your likelihood of developing Alzheimer's disease. Before testing, ask yourself if you really want to know...

• Take omega-3 supplements. Use either fish oil or algae (vegan). Aim for at least 500 mg of EPA and DHA combined, perhaps significantly more.

• Check your omega-3 levels. This can be done with a simple finger stick from a kit that you can order online (without a doctor's order). If your levels are low, increase your DHA and EPA consumption.

• Use a NAD booster to increase your energy and fight aging. Options include nicotinamide riboside (NR) 300 mg/day or nicotinamide mononucleotide (NMN) 250-1000 mg/day.

• Drink exogenous ketone esters in the morning to increase your focus, protect your brain, and possibly boost your athletic performance.

• Try cryotherapy. It decreases inflammation, improves vigor, and it may be anti-aging. The super-cold rooms are probably easier than ice baths. Try them for a few weeks and see how you feel.

• Red light therapy (RLT). Go to a wellness center, dermatologist, or medical spa and try a course of RLT. It will reduce wrinkles, boost skin collagen, help you recover from injuries, and treat scars. Microneedling and intense pulsed light (IPL) will increase your skin collagen and make you look younger.

• Most of the immune-boosting suggestions in this book will probably help protect you from respiratory viruses like COVID-19. In addition to following routine precautions like handwashing and distance, you want to do what you can to strengthen your immune system. In particular, sleep, zinc, and garlic are effective with other similar viruses and will likely reduce your risk of infection from COVID-19.

Don't:

• Skimp out on sleep with the plan of catching up on the weekend. That doesn't work. Missing even one night of sleep appears to have a long-term impact including decreased resistance to infection.

• Assume that you only need 4-5 hours of sleep. It turns out that less than 1% of the population does well with that little sleep. If you think you're one of those people - you're wrong. Sleep deprivation increases your risk of death, impairs your athletic and work performances, and ages you.

• Use sleeping pills. They don't give you quality sleep and they appear to increase your risk of death.

• Give up on treatment for depression because you tried an antidepressant or two without benefit or because you suffered a side effect from your oral antidepressants. There are always other options including ketamine, ECT, cognitive behavioral therapy, or other oral medications.

• Assume that you can't have depression because you're a successful athlete, lawyer, politician, or executive. You can be depressed and have a powerful career. If you're worried you're depressed, go for an evaluation.

• Smoke. Smoking ages you, disrupts your sleep and increases your risk for heart disease, cancer, and stroke. Did I mention that smoking ages you?

• Live near major roads, chemical or manufacturing facilities, or other contaminated places. Chemicals and heavy metals will age you, shorten your telomeres, and increase your risk of cancer and Alzheimer's disease.

• Expose yourself to radiation and excessive sun. Minimize X-rays and seek alternatives to CT scans (like an MRI or ultrasound). Avoid prolonged sun exposure in the afternoon, wear protective clothing, and use mineral-based sunscreens.

- Drink sugary drinks like soda or fruit juice. I know, fruit juice is made from fruit. Unfortunately, it is loaded with fruit sugar and lacks fiber and many nutrients.

Let me share one final tip that will keep you young, improve your mood, and help you sleep at night: volunteer and help those in need.

Cheer up seniors at a nursing home. Read to kids at the local library. Volunteer with your religious organization. Lend a hand (paw?) at the animal shelter. Drive an elderly person to their medical appointments. Feed the homeless. Start a charitable foundation. Clean up a neighborhood park or beach. Mentor disadvantaged youth. The options are endless and your community needs you.

When you give back, you create a life worth living. We all want more healthy time on this Earth. But, we also want to make sure that our time is meaningful.

Giving back is good for you and your community. Strong bonds with other people are anti-aging. Your social ties keep you young (yes, there is actually scientific evidence for this). Helping others will improve your sleep and protect your telomeres. Volunteering is a great way to enhance the quality of life and reduce symptoms of depression. It is truly a win-win.

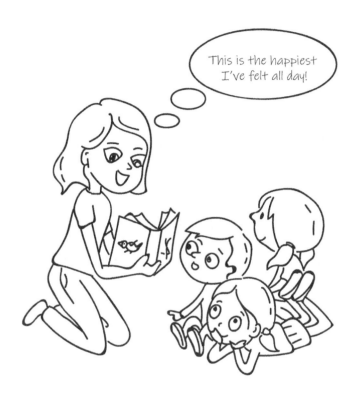

Thanks to medical wellness techniques like the ones mentioned in this book, some people will live much longer, healthier lives. Unfortunately, not everyone knows what to do. Please go out and share the gift of health, gratitude, and kindness with society.

We're all in it together.

(Now, go out there and eat some broccoli!)

It is my hope that *Why Doctors Skip Breakfast* will help you enjoy a longer, healthier, and more meaningful life.

If you found this book useful, please tell your friends and write a nice review on Amazon or wherever you purchased the book. As an independent author, I depend on your support.

If you'd like to share your success stories or give constructive feedback about the book, please contact me directly through my website at www.gregorycharlopmd.com. You can also reach me on Facebook and LinkedIn.

I am available for in-person or telemedicine consults for a limited number of new patients.

Thanks for reading and I wish you limitless health and happiness,

Gregory Charlop, MD

About the Author

Gregory Charlop, MD, is an award-winning physician, author, speaker, and aging expert.

Known as the anesthesiologist to the stars, Dr. Charlop is one of the most sought-after physicians in California.

After training at Stanford and UCLA, Dr. Charlop built a career attending to some of the most complex patients in the San Francisco area. He's spent years on the front lines of healthcare, treating adults and children with uncontrolled pain and complicated medical issues.

Now, he's brought his talents to Beverly Hills and Hollywood. Celebrities and executives fly in from all over the country for plastic surgery under his expert care.

An authority in wellness and advanced nutrition, Dr. Charlop is now sharing his expertise with the world. He's the author of *Why Doctors Skip Breakfast: Wellness Tips to Reverse Aging, Treat Depression, and Get a Good Night's Sleep.* The workbook for *Why Doctors Skip Breakfast* will be available in June 2020.

Dr. Charlop is the founder of an elite wellness and anti-aging clinic in Beverly Hills where he sees athletes and high-achievers by special appointment. His ketamine clinic for depression is available to a limited number of patients by exclusive arrangement.

To make a telemedicine wellness appointment or to discuss speaking engagements, contact Dr. Charlop through his website, www.GregoryCharlopMD.com.

References

To make *Why Doctors Skip Breakfast* easier to read, I intentionally omitted footnotes and excessive references to studies in the body of the text. However, everything in the book is based on rigorous scientific data. This chapter is dedicated to those who'd like to learn more about the research underpinning the book.

I divided the further reading into sections. We begin with other books on similar topics. All these books are well-written and easy to read. I hope you'll read them all. Next, I have a list of websites. Some have useful nutrition information and others are for products mentioned in the book. Finally, we have published research articles and medical advisories divided by topic.

Books

Sinclair, David. *Lifespan: Why We Age and How We Don't Have To.* Atria Books, 2019.

Bredesen, Dale. *The End of Alzheimer's: the First Program to Prevent and Reverse Cognitive Decline.* Penguin Group USA, 2017.

Walker, Matthew. *Why We Sleep: Unlocking the Power of Sleep and Dreams.* Scribner, an imprint of Simon & Schuster, Inc., 2017.

Greger, Michael. *How Not to Die: Discover the Foods Scientifically Proven to Prevent and Reverse Disease.* Flatiron Books, 2015.

Bubbs, Marc. *Peak: The New Science of Athletic Performance That is Revolutionizing Sports.* Chelsea Green Publishing, 2019

Blackburn, Elizabeth. *The Telomere Effect: A Revolutionary Approach to Living Younger, Healthier, Longer.* Grand Central Publishing, 2018.

Websites

https://nutritionfacts.org/
Run by Dr. Greger, author of *How Not to Die*, this site has tons of useful (and somewhat obscure) information about the health value of different foods and herbs. I check it all the time. His material is geared towards the general public.

https://www.cdc.gov/
The CDC is the definitive source of information about the Coronavirus. Go here directly for the latest updates about disease epidemics and skip the misinformation commonly found in the popular press.

https://aasm.org/
The American Academy of Sleep Medicine is a great reference for those interested in learning more about sleep.

https://peterattiamd.com/
A physician, longevity expert, and podcaster, Dr. Attia shares tons of useful information about nutrition and technology. His material is a little more complex.

https://www.dexcom.com/
Dexcom manufactures one of the best continuous glucose monitors (CGMs)

https://www.medtronicdiabetes.com/treatments/continuo us-glucose-monitoring
Medtronic also produces continuous glucose monitors

https://omegaquant.com/
OmegaQuant manufactures a device that will measure your red blood cell omega-3 levels with a finger prick. No prescription needed.

Scientific Papers and Alerts
[Author's note: Yes, I am using non-standard formatting for some of the journal article citations. I am leading with the article's title to make it easier for you to decide which ones you want to read.]

Depression
https://aeon.co/essays/the-evidence-in-favour-of-antidepressants-is-terribly-flawed
(Great article by Aeon about interpreting studies on antidepressants. Highly recommended.)

https://www.sleepfoundation.org/articles/depression-and-sleep
(A nice article about depression and sleep from the National Sleep Foundation)

A brief diet intervention can reduce symptoms of depression in young adults - A randomized controlled trial.
PLoS One. 2019 Oct 9;14(10):e0222768

For Individuals with Obstructive Sleep Apnea, Institution of CPAP therapy is Associated with an Amelioration of Symptoms of Depression which is Sustained Long Term.
J Clin Sleep Med. 2007 Oct 15; 3(6): 631–635.

Cognitive-behavioral therapy for adolescent depression: a meta-analytic investigation of changes in effect-size estimates.
J Am Acad Child Adolesc Psychiatry. 2007 Nov;46(11):1403-13.

Clinical effectiveness of individual cognitive behavioral therapy for depressed older people in primary care: a randomized controlled trial.
Arch Gen Psychiatry. 2009 Dec;66(12):1332-40.

Depression and telomere length: A meta-analysis.
J Affect Disord. 2016 Feb;191:237-47.

Zinc in depression: a meta-analysis.
Biol Psychiatry. 2013 Dec 15;74(12):872-8.

Zinc supplementation augments efficacy of imipramine in treatment resistant patients: A double blind, placebo-controlled study
J Affect Disord. 2009 Nov;118(1-3):187-9.

Effects of Social Support and Volunteering on Depression Among Grandparents Raising Grandchildren.
Int J Aging Hum Dev. 2016 Oct;83(4):491-507.

A psychology of the human brain–gut–microbiome axis
Soc Personal Psychol Compass. 2017 Apr; 11(4): e12309.

Ketamine

Ketamine for Depression, 4: In What Dose, at What Rate, by What Route, for How Long, and at What Frequency?
J Clin Psychiatry. 2017 Jul;78(7):e852-e857

A randomized trial of an N-methyl-D-aspartate antagonist in treatment-resistant major depression.
Arch Gen Psychiatry. 2006 Aug;63(8):856-64.

Efficacy of intravenous ketamine for treatment of chronic posttraumatic stress disorder: a randomized clinical trial.
JAMA Psychiatry. 2014 Jun;71(6):681-8.

Preemptive analgesia with Ketamine for Laparoscopic cholecystectomy
J Anaesthesiol Clin Pharmacol. 2013 Oct-Dec; 29(4): 478–484.

Intravenous Ketamine Infusions for Neuropathic Pain Management: A Promising Therapy in Need of Optimization.
Anesth Analg. 2017 Feb;124(2):661-674

Ketamine Infusions for Treatment Refractory Headache.
Headache. 2017 Feb;57(2):276-282.

Ketamine for Social Anxiety Disorder: A Randomized, Placebo-Controlled Crossover Trial.
Neuropsychopharmacology. 2018 Jan;43(2):325-333.

Ketamine as treatment for post-traumatic stress disorder: a review.
Drugs Context. 2019 Apr 8;8:212305.

Antidepressant efficacy of ketamine in treatment-resistant major depression: a two-site randomized controlled trial.
Am J Psychiatry. 2013 Oct;170(10):1134-42.

Rapid and longer-term antidepressant effects of repeated ketamine infusions in treatment-resistant major depression.
Biol Psychiatry. 2013 Aug 15;74(4):250-6.

A systematic review and meta-analysis of randomized, double-blind, placebo-controlled trials of ketamine in the rapid treatment of major depressive episodes.
Psychol Med. 2015 Mar;45(4):693-704.

Aging medicine

https://www.scientificamerican.com/article/cancer-research-points-to-key-unknowns-about-popular-antiaging-supplements/
(Thought-provoking Scientific American article about the safety of NAD boosters)

Association of Cardiorespiratory Fitness With Long-term Mortality Among Adults Undergoing Exercise Treadmill Testing.
JAMA Netw Open. 2018 Oct 5;1(6):e183605.

Differential effects of endurance, interval, and resistance training on telomerase activity and telomere length in a randomized, controlled study.
Eur Heart J. 2019 Jan 1;40(1):34-46.

Avoidance of sun exposure is a risk factor for all-cause mortality: results from the Melanoma in Southern Sweden cohort.
J Intern Med. 2014 Jul;276(1):77-86.

https://www.uwhealth.org/health/topic/special/radiation -exposure-risks-and-health-effects/abl0600.html
(Nice article from the University of Wisconsin about radiation)

https://www.mayoclinic.org/diseases-conditions/periodontitis/symptoms-causes/syc-20354473
(Useful article from the Mayo Clinic about periodontal disease)
Periodontal diseases and adverse pregnancy outcomes.
J Obstet Gynaecol Res. 2019 Jan;45(1):5-12.

The Association between Meditation Practice and Job Performance: A Cross-Sectional Study.
PLoS One. 2015; 10(5): e0128287.
https://www.theguardian.com/lifeandstyle/2016/nov/28/ breakfast-health-america-kellog-food-lifestyle
(Eye-opening article from The Guardian about how lobbyists made breakfast the "most important meal of the day")

Intermittent fasting confers protection in CNS autoimmunity by altering the gut microbiota
Cell Metab. 2018 Jun 5; 27(6): 1222–1235.e6.

https://osher.ucsf.edu/patient-care/integrative-medicine-resources/cancer-and-nutrition/faq/cancer-and-fasting-calorie-restriction
(Great article by UCSF about cancer, chemotherapy, and fasting)

Abstract 11123: Intermittent Fasting Lifestyle and Human Longevity in Cardiac Catheterization Populations
Circulation. 2019;140:A11123

Caloric restriction improves health and survival of rhesus monkeys.
Nat Commun. 2017 Jan 17;8:14063.

Daily Fasting Improves Health and Survival in Male Mice Independent of Diet Composition and Calories.
Cell Metab. 2019 Jan 8;29(1):221-228.e3.

3-Hydroxybutyrate Regulates Energy Metabolism and Induces BDNF Expression in Cerebral Cortical Neurons
J Neurochem. 2016 Dec; 139(5): 769–781.

https://ghr.nlm.nih.gov/primer/howgeneswork/epigenome
Nice summary of epigenetics from the NIH

https://youtu.be/AvBoq3mg4sQ
Fun video about epigenetics on YouTube

Epigenetic alterations in longevity regulators, reduced life span, and exacerbated aging-related pathology in old father offspring mice.
Proc Natl Acad Sci U S A. 2018 Mar 6;115(10):E2348-E2357.

Targeting senescent cells: approaches, opportunities, challenges.
Aging (Albany NY). 2019 Nov 30;11(24):12844-12861.

Exercise and the aging immune system
Ageing Res Rev. 2012 Jul;11(3):404-20.

Sleep

Sleep Health: Reciprocal Regulation of Sleep and Innate Immunity.
Neuropsychopharmacology. 2017 Jan;42(1):129-155.

The sleep-wake cycle regulates brain interstitial fluid tau in mice and CSF tau in humans.
Science. 2019 Feb 22;363(6429):880-884.

Disruption of the sleep-wake cycle and diurnal fluctuation of β-amyloid in mice with Alzheimer's disease pathology.
Sci Transl Med. 2012 Sep 5;4(150):150ra122.

Delaying Middle School and High School Start Times Promotes Student Health and Performance: An American Academy of Sleep Medicine Position Statement.
J Clin Sleep Med. 2017 Apr 15;13(4):623-625.

Evening use of light-emitting eReaders negatively affects sleep, circadian timing, and next-morning alertness
Proc Natl Acad Sci U S A. 2015 Jan 27;112(4):1232-7.

Shift work and the risk of cardiovascular disease. A systematic review and meta-analysis including dose-response relationship.
Scand J Work Environ Health. 2018 May 1;44(3):229-238.

Shift Work: Disrupted Circadian Rhythms and Sleep-Implications for Health and Well-Being.
Curr Sleep Med Rep. 2017 Jun;3(2):104-112.

Sleep and Elite Performers

https://practicalneurology.com/articles/2019-mar-apr/sleep--elite-athletic-performance
(Great article about sleep and athletic performance by Dr. Kutscher from Stanford University)

Sleep-disordered breathing, hypertension, and obesity in retired National Football League players.
J Am Coll Cardiol. 2010 Oct 19;56(17):1432-3.

Red light and the sleep quality and endurance performance of Chinese female basketball players.
J Athl Train. 2012 Nov-Dec; 47(6):673-8.

IOC consensus statement: dietary supplements and the high-performance athlete.
Br J Sports Med. 2018 Apr;52(7):439-455.

Wellness techniques to guard against the coronavirus and infections

The effectiveness of high dose zinc acetate lozenges on various common cold symptoms: a meta-analysis.

BMC Fam Pract. 2015 Feb 25;16:24.
https://www.ucsf.edu/news/2015/08/131411/short-sleepers-are-four-times-more-likely-catch-cold
(Important article from UCSF showing how sleep protects against the common cold)

Behaviorally Assessed Sleep and Susceptibility to the Common Cold.
Sleep. 2015 Sep 1;38(9):1353-9

Aged Garlic Extract Modifies Human Immunity.
J Nutr. 2016 Feb;146(2):433S-436S.

Evaluation of the efficacy of *Lactobacillus plantarum* HEAL9 and *Lactobacillus paracasei* 8700:2 on aspects of common cold infections in children attending day care: a randomized, double-blind, placebo-controlled clinical study.
Eur J Nutr. 2020 Feb;59(1):409-417

Zinc Acetate Lozenges May Improve the Recovery Rate of Common Cold Patients: An Individual Patient Data Meta-Analysis.
Open Forum Infect Dis. 2017 Apr 3;4(2):ofx059.

Exercise and Respiratory Tract Viral Infections
Exerc Sport Sci Rev. 2009 Oct; 37(4): 157–164.

Made in the USA
Coppell, TX
29 May 2020